THE HEALING POWER OF THE
PINEAL GLAND

Exercises and Meditations to Detoxify, Decalcify, and Activate Your Third Eye

CRYSTAL FENTON

T0020726

ULYSSES PRESS

Published by:
Ulysses Press
PO Box 3440
Berkeley, CA 94703
www.ulyssespress.com

ISBN: 978-1-64604-340-8
Library of Congress Control Number: 2021946578

Printed in the United States by Kingery Printing Company
10 9 8 7 6 5 4 3 2 1

Acquisitions editor: Casie Vogel
Managing editor: Claire Chun
Project editor: Renee Rutledge
Editor: Anna Embree
Front cover design: David Hastings
Interior design: what!design @ whatweb.com
Layout and production: Jake Flaherty, Yesenia Garcia Lopez
Interior images: © elenabsl/shutterstock.com

PLEASE NOTE: This book has been written and published strictly for informational purposes, and in no way should be used as a substitute for consultation with health-care professionals. You should not consider educational material herein to be the practice of medicine or to replace consultation with a physician or other medical practitioner. The author and publisher are providing you with information in this work so that you can have the knowledge and can choose, at your own risk, to act on that knowledge. The author and publisher also urge all readers to be aware of their health status and to consult health-care professionals before beginning any health program.

THE HEALING POWER OF THE PINEAL GLAND

To the divine timing of the universe, always bringing us to the right place, right when we need to be, cultivating expansion, consciousness, and receptivity to the flow of life.

TABLE OF CONTENTS

INTRODUCTION

As human beings, we are all interconnected by our shared quality of duality: the relationship between our physicality and our spirituality. Our physical selves—the body and the brain—are based in science and anatomy. Our spiritual selves, on the other hand, rely on the energetic state of our existence along with the wisdom found within our hearts.

The purpose of this book is to guide you in learning how to harness the healing power of the pineal gland, which connects with the activation of your third eye chakra. Your third eye chakra, known in Sanskrit as the *ajna chakra*, lies in the space directly between your eyebrows. The pineal gland and the third eye chakra are bound forces, acting as separate portals that work together to activate your awakening of hyperawareness, consciousness, and enhanced clarity of intuition.

In researching and writing this book, I conducted multiple interviews with a range of experts in the health, sleep science, and wellness worlds. This research enhanced my awareness and understanding of the pineal gland and how it connects with the third eye chakra, along with the powerful nature of the human body, its energetic fields, and its own internal healing capabilities.

Holistic Healing to Unlock Your Ultimate Potential

The human body is a system of constantly moving parts; when these parts work in tandem, this ensures optimum functionality. Stress, toxins, congestion, you name it—all of these factors act as obstacles that can manifest physically within the body. And these issues can bring with them negative effects that hinder the clarity of our minds and intuitive abilities.

With this in mind, adopting a holistic approach to caring for ourselves, utilizing self-care practices that encompass mind, body, and spirit, is essential on a daily basis. Especially in our modern environment where time is precious and many external challenges exist, preserving and protecting the energy with which we present ourselves to the world is critical. Also imperative is nurturing and managing our internal thoughts, feelings, and aura in a manner that is reflective of and conducive to how we coexist with challenges or with chaos we cannot control.

While we can't always control or change circumstances or situations in the outside world, we can take the reins in how we handle and process our internal emotions, responses, and actions. The power of the mind is stronger than the physical power of the body.

Activating Chakra Energy

Everything is energy—including you. Our essence extends beyond our physical bodies into vibrational vortexes that radiate outward. The energy centers that exist within these vortexes are known as chakras. The chakras are located along the spinal column, ascending from bottom to top. This corresponds with both physical and spiritual alignment. As the chakras flow upward in a vertical line, our spiritual energy ascends in the same manner, as our neck, head, joints, and spinal column vertically stack upward.

It is widely believed that there are seven chakras, each with a corresponding color:

Muladhara
the root chakra, red

Svadhisthana
the sacral chakra, orange

Manipura
the solar plexus chakra,
yellow

Anahata
the heart chakra,
green

Vishuddha
the throat chakra, blue

Ajna
the third eye chakra,
blue-purple or indigo

Sahasrara
the crown chakra,
violet or white

Think of the chakras as revolving doors that connect your inner being with the physical world that surrounds you. Consider the third eye chakra like a peacock: when it is activated and conscious, you see the world, internally and externally, in full, expansive clarity, similar to how the feathers of a peacock open and expand. Now, you are open and receptive, with clear, focused attention on all the vivid colors, sensorial experiences, and tactile elements that surround you. Conversely, when this third eye chakra is blocked, you can feel stuck, lethargic, and muddled—almost as if everything that exists within and around you is unmoving and blurred, like when a peacock's feathers are blocked and unable to expand fully into their potential.

While the third eye chakra is directly associated with and connected to the pineal gland, all of the other chakras can also have an impact on this gland and its function. Although our understanding is that people have seven chakras, it may be helpful to think of only six of them as residing within the physical body while the seventh, the crown chakra, resides just off of or above the body, acting as a connection point with the divine.

This means that the crown chakra, which is the highest chakra, can flow its source energy, or energy that emits from both our spiritual and physical selves, only in an upward vortex. Located directly below the crown chakra is the third eye chakra, where our pineal gland resides. The third eye chakra, the throat chakra, the heart chakra, the solar plexus chakra, the sacral chakra, and the root chakra all contain both front and back vortexes from which energy can flow and radiate.

Think of your pineal gland as the connection point for the vertical line of energy moving upward through your body, as well as for the flows up and down, left to right, and front to back from your body's multidirectional energy portals. The pineal gland is the final portal before the upward flow of energy to the connection between the crown chakra and the divine, making the pineal gland of great importance in both our physical and spiritual selves.

We will explore the chakras more fully in Chapter 2.

My Journey

Both my personal life and my professional life as a yoga instructor, freelance writer, and journalist center around health, wellness, balance, and helping or being of service to others. This, however, wasn't always the case.

Years ago, I was spiraling into a cycle of negativity. This negative trajectory was the culmination of a pair of traumatic shifts and life changes: a devastating breakup when I had been anticipating an engagement, and a physically and emotionally toxic job and office environment that had cumulatively increased in stress as the years progressed.

Each day, I woke up feeling anxious and off-kilter. This was a harmful combination that crept into and ate away at my creativity, an essential part of my job at a fashion and beauty magazine.

But as the saying goes, everything happens for a reason—even if it doesn't feel like it at the time. These circumstances eventually helped me move toward my true path. Workday and office stress propelled me into deepening my yoga practice. As a coping mechanism to quell the anxiety of a fast-paced, high-pressure environment, I started practicing yoga daily and eventually found my way into a teacher training program.

This yoga practice—uniting the physical body with the emotions and feelings of the mind and the spirituality of the soul—began as a stress-relieving activity and a way to process my grief over the ending of a relationship with the man I thought I would marry. It allowed me to mourn the loss of the future life I had pictured while opening me up to new beginnings, opportunities, and paths.

With my commitment to self-care—practicing yoga, meditation, and mindfulness daily, along with tending to my physical and emotional needs—came a sense of clarity, awakening, and awareness. Emerging from the fog of negativity was like bursting out of a cloud—suddenly, I could see the world in clear, colorful details and envision a positive future.

This propelled me to become a certified yoga instructor and go freelance, something that had previously been too unknown and scary for me to dive into. My creativity, which I took pride in while simultaneously feeling a shortage of, was also awakened, as was my ability to intuit the energy of people and situations.

This is what is often known as the awakening of the third eye chakra: your ability to perceive is heightened, allowing you to "read the room," or discern the aura and energy of events and people. Also activated is an empathetic nature, compelling you to bring service to the world and heal and help others, along with cultivating an enhanced, hyper-focused awareness and level of consciousness.

Your Journey

Now for the good news: you, too, have this same amazing energy within you, waiting to be unleashed into the world. As we move through the following chapters, we'll explore the intricacies of the pineal gland and how to work with it for optimum health, along with how to use mindful, meditative practices and energy-activating exercises to unlock and tap into the power of the third eye chakra.

By learning how to treat, heal, and balance these elements of the mind, body, and spirit, we can create the shifts needed to expand into our fullest potential. Practice the energy-activating exercises that follow with your whole heart, mind, and body. Once the power of your pineal gland and third eye chakra are activated and elevated, watch the clarity and intuitive nature of your new sense of self and state of being elevate your life. Let the journey begin!

CHAPTER 1
THE PINEAL GLAND AND THE POWER OF SLEEP

Circadian Rhythms and Melatonin

The pineal gland is a small yet mighty part of your body. About the size of a grain of rice or a pea, this small, pine cone–shaped gland impacts many elements of your life, from how you make decisions to your perception of reality. Located near the center of the brain and aligned with the midpoint between your eyebrows, the pineal gland's primary responsibility is to produce one of the most influential hormones found in the body: melatonin.

You've likely heard of melatonin, one of the most popular wellness supplements around. A key element to healthy sleep, this hormone regulates the flow of the sleep-wake cycle through both seasonal and circadian cycles.

The brain produces melatonin in response to darkness. This hormone is an essential element in our sleep and sleep quality. Think of the pineal gland's job as that of supervisor, overseeing the command center that controls our sleep quality–perhaps the most important and influential element in our overall physical health and emotional well-being.

Not everyone is aware that the pineal gland is separate from two of the more commonly known command-center glands: the pituitary and the hypothalamus. The pituitary gland is also small, referred to as the master gland due to the fact that it controls the activity of most other hormone-secreting glands. The release of hormones from the pituitary gland is controlled by the hypothalamus, a part of the brain that controls many other functions in the body.

The pineal gland works in harmony with the hypothalamus. The hypothalamus regulates bodily functions such as hunger, thirst, sexual desire, and our biological clock. The pineal gland also manages biorhythms within the body, as we will explore later. Because of its alignment with the midpoint between our eyes, the pineal gland is linked with our third eye chakra. The pineal gland is also thought to contain photoreceptors similar to those found in our eyes. These photoreceptors are activated by light signals transmitted from our eyes.

Because the pineal gland is considered to potentially play a large role in almost every aspect of human function, it must be in optimum health for our bodies and minds to be at their peak levels of performance. The pineal gland is immersed in cerebrospinal fluid. Fluoride from water or pesticides tends to accumulate at higher levels within the pineal gland than in any other part of the body. This can potentially lead to calcification, or hardening, which may hinder or impair the pineal gland's ability to produce melatonin.[1] In fact, the pineal gland has the highest rate of calcification, or development of calcium spots, of any organ.

In addition to producing melatonin, the pineal gland also releases melatonin's partner, serotonin. The production cycle of these hormones is fairly simple: During the day, when there's sunlight, the pineal gland produces serotonin. In darkness or under moonlight, the pineal gland produces melatonin. Both are chemically derived from the alkaloid substance tryptamine and synthesized within the pineal gland. These can then be released into the blood and perhaps also into the cerebrospinal fluid, or brain fluid.

Unlike most other areas of the brain, the pineal gland doesn't have the blood-brain barrier to give it full protection from the rest of the body. The pineal gland receives a significant level of blood flow, second only to the kidneys. The location of this gland deep within the brain may be a signifier of its importance. Hence the pineal gland's role both as the connection between the spiritual realm and our physical existence and as the bridge to the awakening of our third eye chakra.

The Science of Sleep

Ah, sleep. The fundamental and sometimes elusive state that regulates our existence. Being unconscious fuels our consciousness, making sleep essential for both our physical and emotional health.

Sleep and your sleep quality are essential for the health of your whole body, from head to toe. The overnight hours are the body's prime time to restore, renew, rejuvenate, and rest. Many of us, however, have trouble falling asleep, staying asleep, or generally getting enough sleep.

---

1   Melinda Ratini, "What to Know About Calcification of the Pineal Gland," WebMD, June 23, 2021 , https://www.webmd.com/sleep-disorders/what-to-know-about-calcification-of-the-pineal-gland.

Our whole-body, holistic health is dependent on sleep. Without adequate rest, the human body cannot run at its optimum functionality, nor can the brain perform its necessary waste elimination.

As we sleep, the body carries out significant cellular repair and rejuvenation, while the brain eliminates harmful wastes and toxins. The nervous system moves into its resting phases, stress hormones drop to their lowest levels, and the immune system resets. Our cognitive and psychological health benefits from the memory processing and cellular renewal that occur during sleep.

When we are lacking in consistent, high-quality sleep, we miss out on the full impact of its deeply restorative powers. In fact, poor sleep quality increases inflammation, a leading cause of biological aging as well as a significant factor in age-related conditions including heart disease, cancer, and neurodegenerative disorders. Without adequate sleep, the body can't function properly. And neither can the brain.

Enter the pineal gland. If this small yet mighty spot in your brain isn't optimized, then your melatonin production likely isn't as good as it could—or should—be. And if melatonin is lacking, then it's likely that your sleep quantity and quality are also not at their best.

How Circadian Rhythms Regulate Your Sleep

As the primary producer of melatonin, the pineal gland plays an essential role in our overall health by controlling and regulating our biorhythms. Biorhythms are internal rhythmic biological processes that help determine and regulate bodily functions and processes.

The most important of these is our circadian rhythm. Commonly known as the sleep cycle, this light-linked rhythm regulates daily sleeping and waking patterns. Circadian rhythms are mental, behavioral, and physical changes that follow a twenty-four-hour cycle. The rhythms respond primarily to light and dark, and they influence the majority of living beings: plants, animals, and even microbes.

Why is this all important? As mentioned in the previous section, sleep ensures that our bodies are happy, healthy, and running at their best. Conversely, a lack of quality (emphasis on "quality") sleep will likely negatively impact everything about our lives, both physical and emotional. Sleep is necessary for keeping our bodies and brains healthy and functioning at their best. Those lacking in sleep may experience poor memory and focus, lowered immunity, or mood changes.

The REM (rapid eye movement) sleep stage, in which the eyes dart back and forth behind the eyelids, activates the sympathetic nervous system, also known as the "fight-or-flight" response to external stressors. In this stage, your pulse, body temperature, breathing, and blood pressure all rise to daytime levels.

The REM stage is thought to help the brain clear out the clutter of information it no longer needs. Those lacking in REM sleep lose this advantage. Practicing sleep-oriented yoga before bedtime is another way to mentally declutter, eliminating tension stored in the body and adding clarity within the mind.

Let's Talk Melatonin and Circadian Rhythms

Melatonin is essential in regulating circadian rhythms. Our bodies maintain these twenty-four-hour cycles in order to function properly. While circadian rhythms sound similar to the idea of a biological clock, they're not the same. But biological clocks, which are an innate, internal regulatory system of life cycles, do operate in all living organisms, acting in part as natural timing devices that influence circadian rhythms.

Both our biological clocks and circadian rhythms can change and adapt, depending on seasonal shifts as well on our bodies' changing needs as we age. Your circadian rhythm also impacts many of your biological processes, including the functioning of your immune system AND your overall physical and mental health.

One of the most important external factors influencing circadian rhythms is exposure to light. Historically, our circadian rhythms were entirely aligned with the cycles of the sun. The human body most naturally rises with the sun in the mornings and relaxes into sleep with the sun's setting in the evening. This, however, was prior to the invention of artificial light and electronic devices.

The Circadian Rhythm and Its Impact on Healthy Sleep

Circadian rhythms are responsible for regulating your sleep-wake cycle. Your brain produces less melatonin during the morning and daytime and more in the evening and at night. When everything is working as it should, it's likely you'll experience increased levels of alertness during daylight hours. Conversely, you'll likely experience increased levels of drowsiness as the evening progresses and bedtime approaches.

An interrupted circadian rhythm can be linked to a disruption in sleep. In turn, this may contribute to sleep disorders such as sleep deprivation, delayed sleep phase disorder, and excessive daytime drowsiness. Delayed sleep phase disorder, also known as delayed sleep phase syndrome or a delayed sleep phase cycle, is simply as it sounds: when a person has sleep that is delayed by two or more hours, this makes it all the more difficult to wake up the next day.

Just as your circadian rhythm plays a vital role in achieving a good night's sleep, a good night's sleep is equally important in regulating and maintaining a healthy circadian rhythm. Any abnormality in the cycle may act as a disorder that can not only ruin your rest but also throw off your body's equilibrium. Modern life—often filled with and ruled by digital devices rather than the natural rhythm and light of the sun—puts us at risk of disrupting the natural flow of circadian rhythms, thereby sabotaging how we function. We will delve into digital detox exercises in Chapter 16, where we discuss the impact of blue light on the pineal gland and its production of melatonin.

But here's a good place to start: make the hour or two before you go to sleep a sacred time when you avoid interaction with your digital devices as much as possible. During this interlude, force yourself to put away your phone—preferably in another room—and power off all of your other digital devices. This includes your TV, tablet, e-reader, and anything else with a screen.

Instead, pick up a book, magazine, journal, or any other form of entertainment that doesn't expose you to the potential harm of blue light emissions. You may also choose to practice a gentle yoga sequence, go for a relaxed walk, or take a bath. . . anything that helps you unwind without electronic connectivity. After all, don't we already spend too much time tethered to screens and constant connectivity in our waking lives? Minimizing screen time may make a significant difference in your sleep patterns and bolster your pineal gland's healing power.

Melatonin Supplements

Let's discuss melatonin and its use as a supplement. While melatonin is produced naturally within the body by our pineal gland, it's likely that you've heard about its availability as a supplement. The level of naturally produced melatonin in the blood is highest at night. This, in turn, helps to naturally facilitate the transition to effective, productive sleep. However, if you feel your melatonin production is lacking naturally, a supplement may be a helpful tool for a better night's sleep. Some research suggests that taking melatonin supplements may be helpful in preventing, treating, and alleviating some of these sleep disorders:

- Delayed sleep phase cycle

- Insomnia

- Jet lag

- Repeated waking

- Trouble staying asleep

- Trouble falling asleep

Melatonin supplements are generally safe for short-term use. One of their benefits is that unlike many other types of sleep medications, especially those requiring a doctor's prescription, you are typically unlikely to become dependent on them. Nor do most people experience foggy next-day hangover effects.

The most common side effects of melatonin supplements include headache, dizziness, nausea, and drowsiness. Other, far less common side effects include short-term depression, mild tremors, mild anxiety, abdominal cramps, irritability, reduced alertness, confusion or disorientation, and abnormally low blood pressure (hypotension).

The use of melatonin supplements can cause daytime drowsiness, so don't drive within five hours of taking a supplement. Melatonin supplements can also potentially interact with various medications such as anticoagulants and antiplatelet drugs, contraceptive drugs, and immunosuppressants. If you're considering taking melatonin supplements, be sure to check with your doctor first.

Increased melatonin production has been reported to improve sleep efficiency, and it has also been noted that certain foods can help with improved melatonin production. While melatonin supplements boost the melatonin-producing function of the pineal gland, if you would rather take a natural route, there are alternatives. To improve and increase the ability of the pineal gland to produce melatonin, try tapping into natural methods of boosting its function, such as eating a healthful diet.

In any efforts to decalcify the pineal gland and clear it of blockages, it's a must to detoxify the gland. This can help to awaken the third eye chakra. Detoxification is especially important because the pineal gland is not protected by the brain-blood barrier, leaving it vulnerable to harmful toxins in the bloodstream.

Fluoride, in its synthetic form, is one toxin that can weaken and otherwise negatively affect the pineal gland as well as other organs throughout the body. Increased fluoride, from toothpaste or tap water or both, can cause the pineal gland to harden, or calcify. This may cause a decrease in melatonin production and disrupt the sleep-wake cycle.

To avoid this from happening, consider completely stopping the use of any toothpaste containing fluoride, which can calcify the teeth or be absorbed into the bloodstream, eventually making its way to the pineal gland. Switching to a fluoride-free formula that utilizes more natural ingredients can help minimize the risks of excess fluoride absorption in the body or buildup on the teeth. Next, switch to using only filtered water both for drinking and brushing your teeth in order to eradicate excess fluoride intake.

To further detoxify the pineal gland, follow the old adage "you are what you eat." Opting for an unprocessed, whole-food diet that excludes as much sugar and dairy as possible and focuses on the power of plants, nature's medicine, can bolster your overall health, including that of your pineal gland. Foods that are plant-based may also help to boost oxygen levels and bolster immune function. Eating and maintaining a balanced, healthful diet that integrates magnesium- and melatonin-rich food can improve and boost the pineal gland's primary function of producing melatonin. Magnesium is thought to help improve sleep and may help alleviate insomnia.

Foods that may assist in better sleep are rich in essential nutrients such as protein, biotin (vitamin B7), selenium, magnesium, and melatonin. These foods include leafy greens, turmeric, tamarind, cacao beans, apple cider vinegar, beets, eggs, fish, nuts such as Brazil nuts, mushrooms such as reishis, cereals, fruits such as kiwis, and germinated legumes or seeds. Some studies have shown that melatonin stimulates many bioactivities, such as antioxidant activity, anti-inflammatory characteristics, immunity boosting, anticancer activity, cardiovascular protection, and anti-diabetic, anti-obesity, neuroprotective, and anti-aging activities.

To further support the elimination of toxins, decalcification, and improved tissue renewal, iodine-rich foods can aid in the removal of heavy metals and fluoride.

Stress and Sleep: A Complex Cycle

Sleep—or the lack of it—and stress often go hand in hand. And stress can be the culprit behind an array of other health issues. Aside from wreaking general havoc on your mind and body, stress can lead to delayed or altered production of the melatonin levels needed for an adequate night's sleep.

Fortunately, there are ways to stop stress in its tracks. A pre-bedtime yoga routine, for example, will help quiet the mind, quell anxiety, and induce the calm, relaxed state needed to drift off into a good night's rest. Other evening routines that quiet the mind include meditation (page 44), journaling (page 89), gratitude practice (page 81), positive affirmations or mantras (page 57), self-care rituals (page 100), and digital detoxing (page 114). As is so often true, if we can unplug and rest, our systems can get a reboot.

Whether it's only perceived or stems from an actual external aggressor, stress manifests in the same physical responses within the body. When your body's sympathetic nervous system is activated, the physical response goes to fight-or-flight mode. Stress causes the body to produce more cortisol, which is the catalyst for the release of pro-inflammatory cytokines. These are proteins that act as messengers between cells. Cytokines regulate functions such as inflammatory response—sometimes stimulating it, sometimes suppressing it.

Some stress, however, is necessary in order for many physical nervous system processes, such as those of the sympathetic and parasympathetic nervous systems, to respond and function appropriately.

A self-care practice can soothe, calm, and release you into an easeful night's sleep. By completing and practicing the activities that follow, you can learn to activate and regulate the function of your pineal gland, thereby awakening your energy and unlocking the chakras, including your third eye chakra. Achieving a higher level of awareness and consciousness through the processes of detoxification and decalcification can lead to a bolstered vibration of your energy and more clarity in your thoughts and intuition. Then you'll be able to fully experience all moments with mindfulness and be present in the now.

CHAPTER 2
AWAKENING, UNLOCKING, AND UNBLOCKING THE CHAKRAS

Exploring Your Energy Vortexes

Aside from its primary responsibility in the production of melatonin, the pineal gland is also linked to the powerful energy center known as the third eye chakra.

The connection between the third eye chakra and the pineal gland is important because they both act as portals to consciousness and clarity of intuition. An activated third eye chakra brings with it wisdom and vivid, focused awareness. When awakened, the third eye chakra can cultivate enhanced insight and vision, along with the ability to connect and transcend into a concentrated state of consciousness.

Chakras, also known as energy centers, act like vortexes. Cohesive, easy energy flow is essential to our health, in both our physical bodies and our emotional responses, and the chakras act as pathways for unleashing our full power and possibility.

Chakras can be traced back to the oldest and most sacred texts of ancient Indian culture in south Asia: the Vedas. These ancient texts were written in the Sanskrit language, and the word "chakra" stems from the Sanskrit word for "disk" or "wheel." Chakras are a key part of ancient Vedic healing practices. In the practice of Ayurvedic medicine, which evolved from the Vedas, any illness, ailment, distress, or congestion to or within the physical body is viewed as an energy blockage rooted in one or more of the chakras.

Each chakra correlates to a color or shades of color. We will learn what these colors mean and why the chakras' energetic fields are directed in an upward motion. We'll explore the unique energy of each chakra, as well how each one is related, directly (as with the third eye chakra) or indirectly, to the pineal gland and its function.

CHAKRA EXPLORATION EXERCISE

Before we delve into the unique intricacies and energies of each chakra, let's explore how the chakras' subtle energies feel.

- Begin by lying down on your back.

- Gently rub your hands together and then softly clap them a few times to activate the power of touch.

- Close your eyes. This will help you tune in to your inner universe and get in touch with your internal, intuitive awareness.

- Place your right hand above the lowest part of your groin area, where the root chakra is located.

- Move your hand slowly away from your body, about a foot or so, and then very slowly bring it back in until you can sense the energy radiating from your body. This may feel prickly for some, soft for others, or soft and calming for others.

- Ask yourself, silently or aloud, questions about this exercise. What does this energy feel like? Does the energy feel soft, prickly, warm, cool, absorbent, calming, or something else entirely? Are there other qualities you can feel in this energy? How far away or close to your body does the energy flow?

- Repeat this process for each of the chakras at their specified locations.

  - Sacral chakra: over your pelvis

  - Solar plexus chakra: over your solar plexus, just below where your ribs part

  - Heart chakra: within the center of your chest

  - Throat chakra: within the direct center of your throat

  - Third eye chakra: within the center of your forehead, right above and between your eyebrows

  - Crown chakra: just above the center of your head

- You may also wish to repeat the entire process a second time with your left hand to see whether anything feels different. Be sure to cleanse and reactivate your hands before doing the second sequence.

- Gently open your eyes, bringing your awareness back into the physical space that surrounds you.

ROOT or MULADHARA CHAKRA

The root chakra, known in Sanskrit as the muladhara chakra, is connected with the color red. In Sanskrit, "muladhara" translates to "root" or "support," and this chakra is thought to be where male sexual energy resides in the body. Located at the base of your spine, this is where your energy is believed to originate from, making it arguably one of the most important chakras.

The root chakra is associated with the element of earth and your sense of smell. This root chakra is connected with your most primal, animalistic nature and your need to survive, and it governs your feet, legs, perineum, and rectum. The root chakra also vibrates the most slowly of all of the chakras.

The root chakra is the center of stability and, therefore, when it's out of alignment, you may feel anxious, nervous, or even dizzy. If it's in overdrive, you can feel stagnant in your most important relationships. Either one of these extremes can feel deeply troubling, making you feel as if your life is being uprooted.

To balance this chakra, focus on grounding. While grounding and being connected to the earth seems simple, it's arguably more complex and complicated than most people believe. Grounding is also the primary challenge for many energy workers and empaths. Being unable to ground ourselves can make it difficult to manifest our desires effectively or quickly. (See page 111 for a grounding exercise.)

Learning to engage both the lower and upper chakras at the same time in order to receive guidance and channel intuition will enable us to understand, integrate, and bring these manifestation visions into embodied form. We'll explore more about the power of manifestation in Chapter 6: The Power of Positive Affirmations and Belief and Chapter 7: Manifesting with the Power of the Moon.

The root chakra is indirectly connected with the pineal gland, but that doesn't mean the energy of this chakra doesn't have an impact on the pineal gland and its function. Because the root chakra literally roots us down into the earth, this chakra is all about physical embodiment, overall vitality and good health, foundational influences, security and safety, and the ability to manifest successfully.

Because the root chakra acts as a base, this center of stability and strength is important in maintaining our balance and sense of alignment, both physically and mentally. Being balanced will stabilize the functions of the physical body and their regulation, including that of the pineal gland. When this chakra is off balance, it can throw the functioning of the pineal gland and other systems out of whack.

EXPLORING YOUR ROOT CHAKRA ENERGY

Tapping into the energy of your root chakra can help connect you with the grounded energy of the earth element.

- Close your eyes and prepare to perform a visualization activity.
- Imagine yourself as an enormous redwood tree, standing high, rooted and embodied in your natural power.
- Feel as if you are tall, sturdy, and grounded in your roots.
- Visualize your feet as embedded in the nutrients of the earth.
- Take ten or more deep breaths, imagining the smell of the earth with each one.
- When you feel ready, gently open up your eyes, bringing your awareness back into the physical space that surrounds you.

SACRAL or SVADHISTHANA CHAKRA

The second chakra is the sacral chakra, or "svadhisthana" in Sanskrit, and it is linked with the color orange. The sacral chakra resides in between the reproductive organs, in the center of your lower abdomen and pelvis. Because of its location, this chakra represents the life force of creative potential, the domain of creation and procreation, along with manifestations of the future. The sacral chakra governs the areas of the reproductive organs, moving from your pelvic bowl up to your navel.

The sacral chakra is associated with the element of water and the sense of taste. Think of it as the opposite of the root chakra—one a source of stability, stillness, and organization; the other a font of fluidity, movement, and change.

The sacral chakra is thought to be the seat of our divine feminine, and this birthplace of creation stems from the hips. This is the space from which men and women alike give birth to everything, from relationships to curiosity to desire to joy to intimacy.

If this chakra is blocked or is spinning without ease, your sense of creative potential becomes blocked. Your vitality and happiness depend on the clarity of this chakra. And because this is the chakra that gives life to creation, any blockage can also hinder the function of the pineal gland and its creation of melatonin. An aligned and well-balanced sacral chakra, on the other hand, brings life force and creative potential, including that of a properly regulated, high-functioning pineal gland.

EXPLORING YOUR SACRAL CHAKRA ENERGY

- Close your eyes and imagine a slow-moving fluid force, like water making its way down a river or lava flowing down the side of a volcano.
- Feel as if you are glowing with the orange flow of the lava or the warmth of the water.
- Visualize yourself moving with fluidity, snaking sensually through the terrain.
- Feel as if you are moving with ease, despite the existence of any obstacles in your path.
- Feel the flowing, fluid energy as you deeply inhale and exhale.
- After ten or more rounds of breath, softly open your eyes, bringing your awareness back into the physical space that surrounds you.

SOLAR PLEXUS or MANIPURA CHAKRA

Located in the center of your torso above your navel, right below where the ribs part, the solar plexus chakra is known in Sanskrit as the manipura chakra. "Manipura" means "lustrous gem," and this is the place from which your energy shines and your sense of self-worth radiates. The solar plexus chakra sits about two finger-widths above the belly button and rules the midsection and the majority of the digestive organs. This chakra is linked with the color yellow.

The solar plexus chakra is the center of confidence and power. This chakra is also related to your motivation, identity, and ego. The solar plexus chakra is correlated with the fire element and your sense of sight, which links it indirectly with the third eye chakra and the pineal gland. The solar plexus chakra is the center of our intuition and decision-making mind. This chakra is where we experience our "gut feelings" and intuitive inner instincts. Science has shown that there may be brain cells in our stomachs, and the gut microbiome is sometimes referred to as a second brain.[2]

When this solar plexus chakra is aligned, well-balanced, and in equilibrium with the other chakras, it allows you to feel capable, confident, and empowered. The solar plexus chakra is the key to both manifestation and humility. The fire element within this chakra provides the physical body with the energy needed to digest ideas (and food) and provide us with self-assurance and motivation to accomplish our goals. Because the solar plexus chakra is the seat of your will and personal power, if it is strong and aligned, you will feel in control of your physical body—including regulation of the pineal gland—and your emotions. If this chakra is weak or off-balance, you may experience confusion and indecision along with chronic fatigue.

EXPLORING YOUR SOLAR PLEXUS CHAKRA ENERGY

- Close your eyes and imagine that you are the sun, shining bright and strong, radiating immense light and heat from your solar plexus chakra.

- Feel this power and the way it radiates and shines.

- Remind yourself that you are source energy, and that your energy expands and allows things to grow.

- Experience the feeling of shining bright light everywhere.

- Enjoy the sensations of this fullness of your bright light and lightness in your sense of being as you breathe in and out, fully and completely.

---

2. "The Brain-Gut Connection," Johns Hopkins Medicine, accessed November 8, 2021, https://www.hopkinsmedicine.org/health/wellness-and-prevention/the-brain-gut-connection.

🕊 After ten or more rounds of breath, softly open your eyes, bringing your awareness back into the physical space that surrounds you.

HEART or ANAHATA CHAKRA

Known in Sanskrit as the anahata chakra, the heart chakra is connected with the color green. This chakra is the center of your body's energy universe and regulates energy flow, much as your physical heart regulates blood flow. This chakra is located next to your physical heart and holds the duality of both heartache and deep love.

This chakra controls your capacity to hold, heal, and help. It is also your center of compassion and empathy. When this chakra is well aligned, you are able to easily and openly emit and receive love. Love is arguably the only force that raises our consciousness to a more elevated state of experience and awareness. The energy of love holds and shares vibrations that impact all the cells in our bodies as well as radiating out to those around us.

The heart chakra is located within the center of your chest and governs the lungs and diaphragm along with the heart, arms, and hands. Because of this, the heart chakra is associated with the air element and the sense of touch. This chakra is related to gratitude, forgiveness, compassion, empathy, love, and healing, which link it to the power of the pineal gland in regulating the melatonin needed for healthy, healing levels of sleep.

The heart chakra is the balance point between the three physically oriented chakras below it and the three spiritually oriented chakras above it. The heart chakra acts as a bridge that links the body and mind, lust and reason, the earthly and the divine. "Anahata" can be translated to "unstuck" or "unwounded." This chakra is the center of balance within us that cannot be shaken.

As the heart chakra is the center through which we heal, restorative energy moves through our arms and hands, allowing us to bring healing to ourselves and others through the power of touch or through energy work such as reiki. The heart chakra seeks and senses the connections and commonalities between physical objects and emotional experiences. This allows the energy of the chakra to move from the heart center and create a place of acceptance, equalizing the elements of transitory feelings and balancing emotions.

A healthy and balanced heart chakra that is in equilibrium closely resembles the loving, conscious energy of the divine, enabling us to thrive in loving relationships. You can use these powers of equanimity to enhance the healing capabilities of the pineal gland and keep it functioning at its best.

EXPLORING YOUR HEART CHAKRA ENERGY

- Close your eyes and visualize a full, lush meadow within a forest.

- Breathe in the vibrancy of the green grass, the smell of the flowers and plants, and the essential oxygen of the rich forest air.

- Feel the healing love of the peacefulness of nature and your surroundings.

- Embrace this loving, sweet energy as you take ten full rounds of deep, complete inhalations and exhalations.

- After ten or more rounds of breath, softly open your eyes, bringing your awareness back into the physical space that surrounds you.

THROAT or VISHUDDHA CHAKRA

The throat—or in Sanskrit, "vishuddha"—chakra is embodied by the color blue and plays a key role in our creativity, communication, and self-expression. This chakra is linked with trust, our voice, and our ability to clearly articulate our thoughts and ideas.

Speaking allows us to convey our inner truth and wisdom, ideas and emotions. By opening up the throat chakra, we can share our truth openly and freely with others.

The throat chakra is located at the larynx and the center of the throat. The throat chakra governs the area from the base of the neck up to the ears. If this chakra is out of balance, there may be issues such as a feeling of being "locked" within the hinge joint of the jaw or other blocks in communication. And when our physical body cannot communicate effectively with the brain and the spirit, the functionality of the pineal gland may be impacted.

If the throat chakra is blocked, we can have a challenging time communicating. Imbalances within the throat chakra can also cause fear or anxiety in speaking and expressing thoughts, a raspy throat or laryngitis, or TMJ (temporomandibular joint disorder). An aligned throat chakra can be bolstered by healing practices such as yoga, neck stretches, lion's breath pranayama breathing practices, sound vibration work, and journaling. You may also place blue chakra stones or crystal gemstones around and on the throat and sides of the neck while practicing yoga, meditation or sound vibration work, or journaling.

EXPLORING YOUR THROAT CHAKRA ENERGY

- Close your eyes and imagine that you are surrounded by the vibrations and sounds of a magnificent symphony.

- Feel the surge of complementary sounds and vibrations moving in synchronized motion.

- "Listen" internally to this orchestra of sound and vibration.

- Take ten or more full rounds of inhalations and exhalations.

- Gently open your eyes, bringing your awareness back into the physical space that surrounds you.

THIRD EYE or AJNA CHAKRA

Correlated with the colors of purple and indigo, the third eye chakra is known in Sanskrit as the ajna chakra. This third eye chakra is important for our openness, imagination, and centeredness, and for the connection between our physical and spiritual selves. Because the third eye chakra is located near the optical nerves, it connects with auras and energy fields, helping us to sense, or "see," the intangible.

The third eye chakra is located between and slightly above your eyebrows and regulates the area from the sinuses up to the top of the head. This chakra is related to your sixth sense, intuition, and light. It brings expanded vision and a wise, clear, and balanced perception both inwardly and outwardly.

In Sanskrit, "ajna" means "to perceive" or "to command," and because it is the last of your embodied chakras, it acts as both the highest and wisest of observation points. Think of the third eye chakra as your highest command center or most elevated state of mind, a place from which to appraise your energy and establish clarity for making key decisions.

The third eye chakra is the only physical spot on the body where your perceptions of duality dissolve. Here, the masculine and feminine energy channels—the pingala and the ida—merge to become a singular unit. Congruously, this is also where the two hemispheres of the brain synchronize and work together to see in-depth patterns and broad views. This is the home of inner knowledge, your imagination, and your higher self.

The third eye chakra has a multitude of capacities, many of which we will explore in greater detail throughout this book. This ajna chakra is of utmost importance for many facets of our being:

- Intuition
- Openness
- Imagination
- Centeredness
- Connection between our physical and spiritual selves
- Auras
- Regulation of biorhythms, including sleep cycles
- Connection with our other chakras, along with the activation of clairvoyance, psychic abilities, intuition, insight, and paranormal perception
- Communion with the intangible

Any blockage to this ajna chakra may manifest in a number of detrimental ways, such as feeling stuck, having a sense of blurry, unfocused malaise, or not being able to see the big picture or other perspectives.

If any of our chakras are off balance or blocked, we can feel stuck. So how do you recalibrate your flow and equilibrium? First, you must assess your alignment. Practice the Chakra Exploration Exercise on page 15 to evaluate the flow of your chakras.

Anytime you feel a lack of intuition or are sad, sluggish, or unable to sleep, it's likely an indicator of a third eye chakra imbalance. In the following chapters, we will explore exercises to correct, restore, and maintain the ajna chakra in order to fully tap into and unleash the healing power of the pineal gland. These will include the integration of mindful practices into your daily life, such as yoga, meditation, healing with crystal gemstones, visualization, the use of herbs and essential oils, intention setting, manifestation, self-care rituals, anointment and moon rituals, digital detoxification, and other activities.

Taking this integrated approach that focuses on holistic healing and chakra alignment allows us to utilize tools that offer alternative frequencies or vibrations, employing the shifts needed to change, redirect, or transform our energy stream to heal the impacted chakra.

Energy is present within us at all times, but much of that energy lies dormant, waiting for us to awaken and activate it. Energy moves more powerfully once it is activated.

Because the third eye chakra is a projecting chakra, visualization and belief also play a significant role. Fortunately, our minds are powerful processors, and the adage "mind over matter" carries much truth. By detoxifying and unlocking the third eye chakra utilizing the following chapters' exercises, you can learn how to harness the energy channels within you to create a healthier, happier, and fully whole life.

According to the principles of Ayurveda, the hours between 10:00 p.m. and 2:00 a.m. are governed by the pitta dosha, which helps to recalibrate and renew all the major systems of your body. The pitta dosha allows the body to digest everything from food to information to emotions. The elemental makeup of pitta consists of fire and water; pitta is commonly translated to that which digests things. In the Ayurvedic tradition, the pitta dosha is what allows us to mentally and biologically digest experiences as well as tangible elements such as food. The pitta dosha acts as a means of achieving both chemical and metabolic transformative experiences. When you skip sleep during this precious four-hour window, you miss out on this vital opportunity to heal.

A good night's sleep is essential to how your body responds to the external world. Other benefits include the following:

- Decreased depression
- Reduced anxiety
- Lowered heart rate and blood pressure
- Increased stress resilience
- Optimism
- Improved memory
- Improved metabolism

EXPLORING YOUR THIRD EYE CHAKRA ENERGY

- ✍ Close your eyes and visualize yourself as the original source energy of light that shines and flows through everything.

- ✍ Invoke the feeling of twinkling, magical stars into your heart and mind. Here you have the gifts of insight and intuition.

- ✍ Feel and breathe into the warm and expansive inner light of your heart and third eye chakra.

- ✍ Breathe fully in and out for at least ten rounds.

- ✍ When you feel ready, softly open your eyes.

CROWN or SAHASRARA CHAKRA

The sahasrara chakra, also known as the crown chakra, corresponds with the color violet or, as it expands upward into unlimited purity of energy, a shade of white. As energy travels upward, both through the body and through the chakras, it becomes an extension of source energy. White contains all colors of light, and the energy within this chakra contains all of the other energies found both within and beyond our chakra vortexes.

The sahasrara chakra is your crown of holy connection to the divine. This chakra sits at the top of the head, where it emanates a bright violet disk of protective light and compassionate energy. "Sahasrara" translates to "thousand fold" and metaphorically describes the multi-petaled lotus residing at the crown. The crown chakra acts as an embodiment of our pure, powerful, and spiritual nature.

When this chakra is open and functioning, you will feel awareness of your connection to God, the divine, or the creator on an intimate level. If this chakra is blocked or inactive, you may feel disconnected and unsure of your relationship to these forces. Answering the call of the spirit is powerful and allows you to say yes to the collective universe.

A balanced, stable, and calm crown chakra connects with the pineal gland by bringing unity, consciousness, awareness, understanding, wisdom, and the firm belief in and intuitive sense of being connected with something deeper than ourselves.

- Close your eyes. Visualize your being as an energy matrix that radiates throughout the universe.

- Feel as if you exist in a state of total awareness and consciousness extending beyond space and time.

- Spend ten or more breaths inhaling and exhaling, envisioning yourself as a bright, pure, white light radiating out into the universe.

- When you feel ready, connected, and at peace, gently open your eyes to your external surroundings.

Channeling the Connection between the Third Eye Chakra and the Pineal Gland

The third eye chakra is a powerful energy center within the body and is connected with the pineal gland. The third eye chakra and the pineal gland are both portals to consciousness and clarity of intuition.

As mentioned, an activated third eye chakra brings with it wisdom and vivid, focused awareness. When awakened, the third eye chakra can cultivate enhanced insight and vision, along with the ability to connect with and transcend into a concentrated state of consciousness.

The chakras are the body's energy vortexes. These energy centers determine how, where, and why energy is flowing within your physical body. The chakras also channel and regulate your etheric body, which is the first layer or aura of the physical body.

How our energy flows controls our health, happiness, and harmony. Understanding, organizing, and improving our energy flow can bolster wellness in all areas of life. The chakras act as doorways to possibility and power.

Just as it is said that the eyes are the windows of the soul, so is the third eye chakra the window to both our intuition and the clarity that the wisdom within our intuition brings us. When this chakra is activated, it's as if your eyes are wide open to all of the energies around you, fully sensing all the colors and sensorial experiences available within the external environment.

Conversely, when the third eye chakra is blocked, you're unfocused, unclear, and unable to sense what is surrounding you. You can exist without an awakened third eye chakra—many people do—but why would you want to shut yourself off from the possibilities that surround you? When you begin to question and wonder about the depths of life and consciousness, it's time to open up and activate this chakra to bring in all the vivid and wondrous elements of life.

Holistic healing is a process that begins from within, connecting the mind with the physical body as well as with a sense of community with others. In the chapters that follow, we will learn to utilize the power of our pineal gland and third eye chakra to regulate and harmonize mind, body, and spirit. Each chapter presents specific activities, exercises, and practices to engage, cleanse, and clarify the third eye chakra.

This guide is meant to bring balance to both your physical body and your emotional mind. Harness the healing power of your third eye chakra and activate the full potential of your pineal gland's power with the activating energy flow exercises and activities in the following chapters.

CHAPTER 3

YOGA PRACTICE FOR BETTER SLEEP

Yoga Sequences and Calming Poses for Sleep

"Yoga does not just change the way we see things;
it transforms the person who sees."

—B. K. S. Iyengar

Yoga is a powerful practice that allows us to transcend beyond merely moving our physical bodies; rather, it connects our physical bodies with our minds and our spirits. Specific yoga poses can have an impact on the pineal gland, especially those asanas, or positions, that work directly with the head, such as inversions.

The word "yoga" is often translated from its Sanskrit origins as a "yoking" or union of the mind, body, and soul. Yoga is an ancient practice dating back thousands of years to its origins in India. Here in the Western world, we often associate yoga with movement and stretching. In the eight limbs (or paths) of yoga, however, asana (the poses) is actually listed as third, rather than first, on the path of a yoga practice.

The Yoga Sutras of Patanjali, the spiritual text of the ancient Indian sage, is associated with the classical format of yoga. Here, yoga is explained as a path of "eight limbs" in which the eight-fold path details guidelines for a purposeful, meaningful life of moral and ethical conduct and self-discipline. Yoga is a practice that is constantly shifting and evolving, changing each time you unroll your mat.

This eight-fold path is called ashtanga—a style of yoga commonly practiced in the West—which translates to "eight limbs." "Ashta" means "eight" and "anga" means "limb." The eight-fold path is a practice to help us become aware of and better our physical health and spiritual nature.

The first four stages are focused on gaining mastery of the body, developing and refining our personalities, and opening up to an energetic awareness of ourselves. All four of these first limbs prepare us for the second half of the journey; the latter four limbs are related to our senses, our minds, and attaining a higher state of consciousness, awareness, and activation of our energetic and spiritual selves.

The eight limbs of yoga are as follows:

1. YAMA: These are guidelines for dealing with ethical standards and integrity. The yamas are focused on our own behaviors and how we conduct ourselves in life.

- **AHIMSA:** nonviolence

- **SATYA:** truthfulness

- **ASTEYA:** not stealing

- **BRAHMACHARYA:** continence

- **APARIGRAHA:** not coveting or not being envious

2. NIYAMA: The second limb is correlated with spiritual observation and self-discipline. Think of regularly practicing poses and meditation or attending church or prayer as examples of putting the five niyamas into daily practice.

- **SAUCHA:** cleanliness

- **SAMTOSA:** contentment

- **TAPAS:** heat or spiritual austerity

- **SVADHYAYA:** study of oneself and sacred scriptures

- **ISVARA PRANIDHANA:** surrender to the divine

3. ASANA: This is the practice of yoga postures in order to develop discipline and the ability to focus and concentrate. The body is viewed as a temple of the spirit, and keeping it in top shape is essential for spiritual growth.

4. PRANAYAMA: Typically translated as "breath control," the breathing techniques in this practice is meant to master the respiratory function while enhancing interconnection of breath, mind, body, and emotion. It is believed that pranayama extends life.

5. PRATYAHARA: This fifth limb is the withdrawal from or transcendence of one (or potentially more) of our senses by consciously moving awareness away from the external world and stimulation that exists outside our bodies. Within this practice we can cultivate detachment, stepping back to look at ourselves internally. One example would be practicing yoga postures with a blindfold or with your eyes closed in order to focus on what's going on inside—rather than outside—yourself at that moment.

6. DHARANA: The sixth limb is concentration or making use of the previous practice of relieving ourselves of outward distractions. Now we can deal with the distractions of the mind to learn how to slow, still, and focus the process of thinking.

7. DHYANA: This seventh limb is contemplation or meditation. Here we have the uninterrupted flow of focused concentration and stillness. This is the ultimate state of having quieted the mind and having few or no thoughts to disrupt the state of hyperawareness without focus.

8. SAMADHI: The eighth limb is ecstasy or bliss. Here, we've reached the point of transcending the self completely, while having activated and become aware of our connection to the divine as well as to the energy and spirit of all living beings.

Say Aum to a Better Night of Sleep

Whether you're a night owl or a morning person, easing into bed with a regular routine—one that includes rolling out a yoga mat—might just help you sleep better. Practicing specific yoga poses as well as the philosophy and concepts of the eight-fold path can help you to cleanse and clarify your pineal gland and third eye chakra. By combining the elements of breath, including chanting the sacred sound of the universe, "Aum," into your practices of mindfulness, yoga, meditation, and self-care, you can raise your energetic vibration. In turn, combining these elements with subtle movements, such as gentle articulations of the spine and integrating slow, calm, clear thinking, we learn and cultivate how to relax, reset, and unwind into the sleeping areas ahead.

Here are some examples of the many ways that yoga can improve your evening routine, leading to a healthy night's sleep:

- Supporting enhanced immune function during the body's overnight repair hours
- Enhancing joint mobility
- Increasing flexibility

- Promoting relaxation
- Calming both the physical body and the mind
- Resetting the nervous system
- Recalibrating your energetic state
- Relieving muscle tension
- Enhancing clarity of mind
- Creating presence in the moment
- Allowing for mindful, focused breathing techniques
- Slowing the mind

Both your mind and body will thank you for heading into a good night's rest feeling loose, limber, relaxed, and calm. Bolster your bedtime routine by allowing the yoga poses beginning on page 32 to lull you into a peaceful, healing night of quality sleep.

Yoga Sequences for Sleep

"Health is a state of complete harmony of the body, mind, and spirit. When one is free from physical disabilities and mental distractions, the gates of the soul open."

—B. K. S. Iyengar

Recalibrate, reorganize, and reset with a restorative sequence of yoga poses created with sleep in mind. Restorative yoga often includes the utilization of props such as bolsters, blankets, blocks, straps, and pillows to provide additional support and stability. Practicing restorative yoga postures and lengthening the amount of time we remain in a position while we focus on the act of breathing can help us open up the areas that unconsciously store tension when our physical bodies responds to stress.

Stress, tightness, and tension often manifest themselves physically in our bodies, particularly within the major joints such as the shoulders, sacroiliac joints, and hips, as well as within the back body in areas such as the hamstrings. In fact, the hips are often referred to as the "emotional junk drawers" of the body, where we unconsciously store tension, while the back and hamstrings are other areas where we can hold tightness. As a result of emotions that we don't want to deal with at the moment, we may place physical stress in the back body, where it can go unseen.

Integrating a restorative yoga practice into your pre-bedtime routine can help clear out clutter–creating both physical expansion and mental openness–in preparation for a restful night's sleep. Additionally, cooling inversions such as putting your legs up a wall help can alleviate insomnia by calming and soothing the nervous system, while reclined twists support the organs of elimination in their overnight detoxification process.

The following postures can be practiced in sequential order or separately—go with what flows and works with your body and mind in the present moment. Say "Namaste" (translated as "the light in me salutes the light in you") to having sweet dreams and a relaxed, restful night of sleep!

1. BALASANA (Child's Pose)

- Start on the ground with knees bent under you and shins pressing into your mat.

- Fold your torso forward, moving the upper body and head as far toward the ground as possible. Visualize your forehead touching the mat in front of you. If desired, add a pillow or block under the forehead.

- Extend your arms forward next to your ears or rest them alongside your body, palms facing up for receptivity or down for grounding.

2. UTTANASANA (Standing Forward Bend)

- Begin by standing with feet parallel, keeping legs as close together as possible.

- Fold forward, hinging from your hip flexors, as if you were going to touch your forehead to your shins.

- Press your heels down, straightening your legs fully while pushing your sit bones upward. Keep a slight bend in your knees if they feel hyperextended.

- Try to move your forehead toward your shins.

- In the rag doll variation, grab your elbows with each opposite hand and allow your torso to sway gently from side to side, moving from the hips.

3. SUPTA VIRASANA (Reclining Hero Pose)

- Start by sitting on your shins. Place a bolster or pillow at the base of your tailbone.

- Separate your ankles; use your hands to roll your calves outward and sit between them.

- If necessary, separate your knees to the width of your hips.

- Lie back onto your bolster or cushion; use another cushion to support your head and neck.

4. SUPTA BADDHA KONASANA (Reclining Bound Angle Pose)

- Begin seated, placing a bolster or pillow below your tailbone.

- Bend your knees into a butterfly pose, placing the soles of your feet against one another.

- Lie back so that your body is on an incline, with your spine resting on the bolster or pillow. Support your head with a rolled-up blanket or additional cushion so it is higher than your heart.

- Allow your knees to open as wide as possible and relax fully into the props.

5. MALASANA (Garland Pose)

- Begin by standing with your legs hip distance apart. Bend your knees, lowering your body into a squat with your toes angled toward the outer edges of the mat.

- Moving from your hips, fold forward, placing your hands on the mat (or on blocks) in between your knees.

- Gently tuck your chin in toward your chest, allowing the crown of your head to relax toward the mat while lengthening the back of your neck, from the base of the skull to the top of the shoulders

- You can place a block or pillow under your head if it does not reach the mat.

6. PASCHIMOTTANASANA (Seated Forward Bend)

- Sit with straight legs extended forward. You can place a block in front of your feet for a deeper stretch.

- Extend your arms up, directly next to your ears.

- Fold forward, hinging from the hips. Reach for your ankles, feet, or the block, depending on how much shoulder stretch you want.

7. SUPTA MATSYENDRASANA (Supine Spinal Twist)

- Lie on your back, bending your knees up toward your chest.

- Place your arms in a cactus shape, similar to a goal post around your ears, pressing the back of your shoulder blades and arms gently down into the mat. Bend your elbows with your forearms parallel to your ears and palms facing upward with fingers outstretched. If you prefer, you may extend your arms out straight with your palms facing upward.

- Drop your bent knees to one side; rotate your head and neck in the opposite direction if desired.

- Hold the pose for several rounds of breath, then switch sides.

8. VIPARITA KARANI (Legs up the Wall)

- Lie on your side next to a wall, placing your tailbone and buttocks as close to the wall as possible.

- Rotate to lie on your back, extending your legs straight up along the wall, with the backs of your legs supported by the wall.

- A rolled-up blanket can be placed on top of your feet or a pillow placed underneath your lower belly can create a deeper sensation of feeling grounded.

9. UTTHITA EKA PADA RAJAKAPOTASANA (Half-Leg Pigeon Pose)

- Start either on your hands and knees or in downward dog position, with your palms and feet planted on the mat and your body extending upward in an upside-down V shape. Bend one knee and bring it forward, placing your shin on the ground at a diagonal angle and lowering your hips, moving toward the ground. You can place a block or pillow under your hip for extra support in order to help you release deeper into the stretch.

- Extend through your elongated back leg to deepen the stretch in your hamstrings.

- Gently walk your hands forward. Lower your elbows and rest your forearms on the mat . You can either rest your head on the mat or prop it up on pillows or blocks.

- Switch legs and repeat.

10. UTTHAN PRISTHASANA (Lizard Pose)

- Start on your hands and knees. Bring your thumbs to touch in the center of the mat.
- Bring one foot forward, placing it directly outside the corresponding hand and wrist. The opposite leg will extend straight back; you have the option to place a pillow under the back knee if needed.
- Stretch the body forward to activate the stretch within your front leg's hip flexors.
- Then push your body back, lengthening and stretching your back hamstring.
- Switch position and repeat on the opposite side.

11. SAVASANA (Corpse Pose)

- Lie down on your back. Use a small cushion or rolled-up blanket to support your neck and head if desired.
- Allow your arms to rest along the sides of your body, palms facing up.
- Splay your legs as wide as is comfortable, with your toes pointing outward and heels facing one another.
- As your eyes close, consciously relax your facial muscles, beginning at your temples and moving down your face, softening your cheeks and jaw.
- Observe internally if there is anywhere you are holding on to muscle tension. Relax and release any tension you find.
- Allow your breath to flow at its natural pace and rhythm.

PRE-PRACTICE AND POST-PRACTICE ACTIVITIES

Make your mat and practice space sacred and energetically designed to promote healing.

- Before and after your yoga practice, whether you're at home or in the studio, cleanse your mat and the areas that surround it.

- Wipe down your mat with an essential oil spray.

- f you wish, light a match and burn sage, palo santo, or another cleansing medium to free the air and space of any stagnant, stuck, negative, old, or lingering energy within the room.

- Gather needed props and put away unneeded ones.

- If desired, light a candle to use later as part of a fire-gazing ritual. (For more gazing rituals, see Chapter 5.)

- Set an intention or prayer for both the beginning and closing of your practice.

- Make each pose an exercise in moving meditation and activation of the physical self by integrating deep, full breaths into your practice.

- You may also wish to intensify the activation of your pineal gland by lightly tapping the space between your brows to awaken the third eye chakra's energy before your movement and flow.

Summary

Combine these yoga postures together in a sequence, or practice them individually. Pair each pose with mindful breathing to clarify and soothe your body and spirit, and to relax and unwind into a peaceful night of sleep.

CHAPTER 4
BREATHWORK TO ADD BALANCE

Breathe, Flow, and Regulate the Nervous System

*"Calm is retained by the controlled exhalation
or retention of the breath."*

—Pantanjali

You may choose to pair pranayama breathwork with your nightly yoga. Or you can do these breathing techniques on their own at any time.

Breath can be our friend or foe, depending on whether it controls us or we control it. How we breathe offers clarity and insight into our current energetic state. While breathing is a subconscious act, one our body does to stay alive, we can transform it into a conscious act by becoming aware of and developing better breathing practices.

The manner in which we breathe plays an integral role in the regulation of the central nervous system. The sympathetic nervous system is often described as generating the fight-or-flight state. The parasympathetic nervous system, on the other hand, generates the "rest and digest" state, which regulates the basic functions of the body and their usual workings. This reveals how the pineal gland can be impacted by the state of our nervous system. When all is well and the body is functioning appropriately, so will the pineal gland. When things are running askew, the pineal gland and its functioning can be derailed by elevated stress or other negative dynamics that may impact melatonin production.

If you find yourself taking shallow, labored breaths (like how you breathe during a strenuous workout), you're likely experiencing an activated, heated sympathetic nervous system. This is linked to your fight-or-flight response.

Conversely, practicing mindful, conscious breathing using deep, slow breaths such as those applied while in corpse pose or during meditation will stimulate the parasympathetic nervous system. This will help ease you into the cooling rest-and-digest state.

Pairing mindful breathing with specific yoga postures can reduce the activation of your sympathetic nervous system. Deep breaths taken in for a count of five seconds, held for a count of two seconds, and released for another count of five seconds can activate your parasympathetic nervous system, reducing the stress and anxiety you may be experiencing.

Focusing on breathing can soothe reactive bodies and minds. This focus creates a calmer state of being by promoting quick recovery from the dramatic fluctuations that nervous systems experience. The breathing practices that follow calm the nervous system as well as contribute to a healthy immune system and optimal respiratory function.

BASIC BREATHING EXERCISE

- Take a moment to check in with yourself. Sit in stillness and observe, without judgment, how each inhalation and exhalation feels. What physical sensations are you experiencing?

- Next, breathe fully in and out, allowing your body to do a complete exchange of outgoing carbon dioxide with incoming oxygen. This anchors your focus to the present moment so you can receive the full benefit of your breathwork.

Within the *The Yoga Sutras of Patanjali,* Patanjali explains the parameters of a proper pranayama practice:

- Inhalation

- Retention

- Exhalation

In other variations of pranayama, there are ways to focus your concentration while you are breathing. For example, you can ask yourself the following questions:

- Am I breathing from my heart center, from the base of my spine, or from my belly?

- How long am I holding on the breath?

- Are the lengths of my inhalations equal to the lengths of my exhalations?

Patanjali also identifies pranayama "that occurs during concentration on an internal or external object." This type of breathwork happens automatically and without conscious effort when we are truly immersed in and focused on a situation, experience, or event. In Sanskrit, this is known as "kevala kumbhaka." It's the easy, unintentional retention of breath that happens when you are in a deeply meditative state or moving with and engulfed in the flow of life.

Putting Pranayama into Practice

Try performing the following pranayama practices before bed. You can do one, all, or a combination that suits your time and needs.

PRANAYAMA PRACTICE 1: ALTERNATE NOSTRIL BREATHING

The following short, simple, effective practice is known as alternate nostril breathing or, in Sanskrit, "nadi shodhana pranayama." This technique can balance energy, either inviting calm or boosting alertness.

- Curl your right ring and pinky fingers into your palm.
- Join your middle and index fingers and point your thumb upright.
- Rest your left hand on your thigh.
- Gently press the extended two fingers against the left nostril to seal it off. Inhale through your right nostril for four counts.
- Close your right nostril by pressing it with your thumb and release the left nostril as you exhale out of it for four counts.
- Inhale through the left nostril for four counts.
- Close the left nostril, open the right, and breathe out of it for four counts.
- Practice this exercise for four to six rounds.

PRANAYAMA PRACTICE 2: CHANTING THE AJNA BIJA MANTRA (AUM)

Sound and vibration can help us work with and rechannel any imbalance in our energy. Our third eye chakra vibrates along with the "sound of the universe," or aum, which is pronounced "ah-oh-em."

- As you inhale to a count of three, combine each count with a syllable.
- There will likely be a short breath retention in between each of the three counts.
- Slowly exhale, expelling out the breath completely.
- Repeat for as many rounds as desired.

PRANAYAMA PRACTICE 3: CHANDRA BHEDANA

This breathing technique—which is also known as the moon-piercing breath—is associated with a cooling, introspective, lunar vibration. The opposite of heated, outward-focused solar energy, the chandra bhedana pranayama offers an ideal balance to the swirling energy of the day, allowing you to breathe with ease into the evening.

- With your right hand, use your thumb to close your right nostril.
- Breathe in through your left nostril, filling your torso with air.
- Seal both nostrils.
- Hold the breath for two to three counts.
- Release the right nostril and slowly exhale.
- Continue the pattern, inhaling only through your left nostril and exhaling only through your right.
- Repeat for twelve rounds.

PRANAYAMA PRACTICE 4: LION'S GATE BREATHING

This powerful practice takes its cues from its namesake, the lion, and is a great tension tamer and stress reliever. It stretches the entire face, including the tongue and jaw, while easing forehead and third-eye tension between the eyebrows.

- Kneel with your buttocks resting on your feet. You can also sit in lion pose (simhasana) if you wish. For lion pose, kneel on the floor, crossing the front of one ankle over the back of the other, feet pointing to the sides. Sit back on the top of the heels, placing your palms against your knees. Splay your fingers open like the sharpened claws of a large feline. Or, sit comfortably in a cross-legged position, crisscrossing your ankles or placing them under your buttocks.

- Place your hands on your knees.

- Straighten your arms and extend your fingers as if they were lion claws.

- Inhale through your nostrils.

- Prepare to exhale. Open your mouth wide and stick your tongue as far out as possible toward your chin.

- As you exhale strongly and sharply through your mouth, make a "ha" sound.

- Concentrate on bringing your drishti, which is your pointed awareness or internal focus, toward your third eye chakra as you exhale.

- Inhale, returning your facial expression to neutral.

- Repeat four to six times. If your ankles are crossed, switch the positioning of your feet halfway through the repetitions.

Summary

Our breath gives us life. Without the breath, we cease to exist. And while breathing is an unconscious act, one that our physical body does on its own for survival, we can use the practice of breathwork patterns to transform it into a conscious act.

By making mindful breathing a regular part of our daily practice, we can learn how to control and regulate the breath. This in turn can lead to improvements in our respiratory and immune functions, as well as bolstering our body's natural healing properties and healthy production of internal responses, including the production and fluid flow of melatonin from the pineal gland.

Altering the length of our breath can also help still the mind, quelling anxiety and soothing the nervous system. Many yogis believe that we are born into this world with a certain number of breaths imprinted on our lifespan. Therefore, if and when we can learn to master how we breathe, lengthening each inhalation and exhalation, we can extend our lifespan.

CHAPTER 5
PUTTING MEDITATION INTO ACTION

Stilling, Slowing, Quieting the Mind

"Sleep is the best meditation."

—the Dalai Lama

Let's face it: we've all likely fallen into the trap of acting as our own worst critic by doubting ourselves. Self-doubt can lead to a host of negative energy, creating a hole that can be hard to crawl out of. And this, in turn, impacts how we present ourselves to the world. So what do you do when you just can't quiet that negative inner voice?

You've probably heard people raving about the benefits of meditation, the simple act of bringing focused awareness to breath while in stillness. Not only do meditation and its corresponding patterns of mindful inhalations and exhalations calm your nervous system, create inner peace, boost brainpower, and enhance focus, but sticking to a consistent practice can improve immune function and overall physical health. And a meditation practice can be done anywhere at any time, with no props required.

Some studies have found that a meditation practice actually produces changes in the brain. This "rewiring" of brain circuits that are involved in regulating emotion is thought to minimize stress and control the fluctuations of the mind.

Other research shows that meditation, including reciting mantras either out loud or silently, can help people increase self-compassion, lessen the extremities of negative thoughts, change patterns of belief, and facilitate the sometimes challenging process of learning how to both forgive ourselves and practice forgiveness toward others.

Meditation can help us avoid going down the rabbit hole of self-criticism, which is especially important to release from before trying to go to sleep at night. If your mind is reeling when your head hits the pillow, it's likely your sleep will be interrupted.

Meditation calms the central nervous system and physical body while relaxing the mind. Coming back to attention on breath halts the process of criticism in its path. By quieting the body, we can calm the mind, leading to the relaxed state necessary to fall—and stay—asleep.

Meditation is known to reduce stress. Regardless of the source, stress manifests in the same physical way, elevating cortisol levels. Lowering stress-related cortisol levels can have a positive impact on our bodies' ability to sleep. We know stress impacts everything in our lives, including our health. It can impair the proper functioning of the nervous system, along with other processes within the body. Along with stress comes any of the following:

- Reduced immunity, leading to susceptibility to illness

- Signs of aging, including graying hair and wrinkles

- Potential weight gain

- Problems sleeping

- Elevated cortisol levels

Interestingly, in some creatures, including humans, stress can also act as a catalyst for its own mitigation, activating the pineal gland to reduce stress's negative effects. One of the possible roles of the pineal gland may be stress reduction. One study found that the pineal gland performs a general stress-reduction role, similar to how the adrenal glands play a central role in maintaining homeostasis within the body, including promoting efficient melatonin production.[3]

The fight-or-flight state produces stress that elevates cortisol levels. The constant chatter within your head is an ever-fluctuating narrative that affects both how you think and how you feel. If you can change this narrative, you can change your responses, actions, and reactions. As meditation lessens the extremities of negative thoughts, we can change patterns of belief and facilitate self-forgiveness.

---

3. Van Wyk and Elizabeth Joy, "Pineal-Adrenal Gland Interactions in Search of an Anti-stressogenic Role for Melatonin," accessed November 8, 2021, https://vital.seals.ac.za/vital/access/manager/Repository/vital:4054?site_name=GlobalView&view=null&fo=sm_subject%3A%22Melatonin%22&sort=sort_ss_title%2F.

In order to harness the power of meditation, consistency is key, as is belief in the power of the practices. Learning how to breathe effectively and adopting a consistent schedule of meditative practices can retrain both the brain and the body.

Meditation allows us to be responsive instead of reactive in challenging situations. Mindfulness and meditation train our entire system to equilibrate and balance, even when we are not actively practicing meditation at the moment in question.

Before training, our brains are scattered with thoughts each second of every day. Remember, however: meditation is not the act of completely sweeping the mind of thoughts. Rather, meditation is the practice of continually bringing the wandering mind back to the breath over and over and over again, with as little judgment and as much compassion as possible.

QUIETING THE MONKEY MIND WITH MEDITATION

In some types of Buddhist meditation, the mind is compared to a drunken monkey that can spiral wildly if and when we let it. The practice of sitting in stillness, quietly, and using breath to tune in within can still our thoughts from spiraling out of control. To perform a mindful moment or a few minutes of a meditation designed to ease and calm this "monkey mindset," try the following exercise:

- Sit comfortably, propped upright by pillows or any other form of soft support if so desired.
- Allow your gaze to focus on a spot in front of your field of vision or away from your periphery line of sight.
- Keep your gaze fixed and focused, yet soft and relaxed.
- Observe if there is anywhere in your body where you are clenching or holding on to tightness. If so, try to relax those areas.
- Start to pay attention to your breath, noticing how it feels to inhale and to exhale.
- As you bring awareness into each inhalation and exhalation, notice the quality of the breath.
- Observe, without judgment, the sensations you are experiencing with each breath.

- Do the inhales feel expansive and open, as if there is an inflation of the lungs, chest, and abdomen?

- Do the exhalations feel like a release, allowing the body to deflate as you expel old air and energy?

- If a thought pops into your head or your mind begins to wander, simply file the thought away as a stray idea to consider again later. Don't judge these thoughts; simply allow them to be what they are and release them.

- When you feel ready, ease out of the exercise by moving slowly out of your seated position. You may choose to write down any thoughts that arose or note how you felt before, during, and after the exercise.

"Many believe meditation is practiced simply to clear the mind. It's not. Meditation trains the mind to 'sit and stay' and focus on the object of meditation. The object could be your breath, a candle flame, a flower, your footsteps, or a yoga pose, for example," says Olivia Mead, founder of YogaShield: Yoga for First Responders and of Yoga for the Conception Journey. "When the mind is trained to be still, the nervous system can feel safe and steady. Only when the nervous system feels safe will it offer energy to other areas besides survival. This is when we start to see skin clearing up, hair becoming healthier, and more effective sleep, which is always the biggest key to holistic health."[4]

Meditation is a powerful process that can help us to slow down and sit in stillness. In turn, this can allow a practitioner to become truly aware and tune in to what is going on for them both emotionally and physically. Being observant and noticing how we feel, with patience and without judgment, is a helpful practice that can be applied to all parts of our lives, well beyond the meditation cushion. We can empower ourselves to make conscious choices about how we treat ourselves, whom we surround ourselves with, and what we put into our bodies.

Putting meditation into action can bring many of the following benefits:

- Inner peace
- Lowered stress levels
- Increased brainpower
- Enhanced focus and awareness
- Improved immune and respiratory function
- Alleviation of anxiety
- Reduced cortisol
- Present state of mind
- Balance in body, mind, and spirit
- Improved mental health
- Regulated blood pressure
- Improved blood circulation

Meditation can help us curate thoughtful responses to problems or have a positive impact on our ability to execute control over difficult situations. If you don't have control of a situation, work on training your mind to either accept the circumstances or be thoughtful about your emotional response to them. A daily gratitude exercise can be combined with your meditation practice to bolster your resilience in the face of challenges.

---

4.   Olivia Mead, phone and email interview, week of May 1, 2021.

THE HEALING POWER OF THE PINEAL GLAND

DAILY GRATITUDE HABIT

Each morning as soon as you wake up, write down three things you are grateful for. Repeat the exercise in the evening right before bed. Follow the practice for a week.

🖎 Monday morning

1. ....

2. ....

3. ....

🖎 Monday evening

1. ....

2. ....

3. ....

🖎 Tuesday morning

1. ....

2. ....

3. ....

🖎 Tuesday evening

1. ....

2. ....

3. ....

Wednesday morning

1. ....

2. ....

3. ....

Wednesday evening

1. ....

2. ....

3. ....

Thursday morning

1. ....

2. ....

3. ....

Thursday evening

1. ....

2. ....

3. ....

Friday morning

1. ....

2. ....

3. ....

🖎 Friday evening

1. ....

2. ....

3. ....

🖎 Saturday morning

1. ....

2. ....

3. ....

🖎 Saturday evening

1. ....

2. ....

3. ....

🖎 Sunday morning

1. ....

2. ....

3. ....

🖎 Sunday evening

1. ....

2. ....

3. ....

After a week, observe if you notice any changes in your emotions. Consider continuing the practice beyond the initial week. It's said that it takes twenty-one days for a habit to become part of your lifestyle!

Mind (and Meditation) over Matter

Along with how we speak to ourselves, what we believe is also important—and words have power. Can practicing guided meditation or reciting mantras and affirmations impact your health? Your mind is far more powerful than you might think!

MANTRA MEDITATION

Choose a positive affirmation, mantra, phrase, or sentence you wish to incorporate into your meditation.

✎ Write it down.

- As your practice breathing in and out, recite this affirmation, repeating it with each round of breath. You can choose to voice the words aloud or repeat them silently within your mind, or do a combination of the two.

Meditation in Action

Take a few mindful moments at the end of each day to sit in stillness, quiet your mind, allow stray thoughts to dissolve, and breathe. If we think and speak the desires and intentions of our hearts into existence, we can make these dreams manifest into actuality. Slowing down and remembering to breathe is one of the most important things we can do for ourselves, and in turn, for others.

CANDLE GAZING (TRATAKA)

The meditation practice of candle gazing opens up the third eye chakra and pineal gland, improving our focus, concentration, and perhaps even our eyesight. It can be combined with focused breathing using inhalations and exhalations that are equal in length.

- Sit in a quiet, dim space where you will be undisturbed.
- Gather your supplies for this exercise: a candle, safety matches, and candleholder to collect excess wax.
- Place your candle in front of you at eye level on a flat, level, stable surface.
- Light the candle.
- Sit in a comfortable position. Use a meditation cushion or pillow if desired.
- Gaze at the candle's flame flickering. Try to keep a fixed gaze on the flame without blinking or fidgeting.
- Envision the flame imprinting its fire into your chakras, fueling the opening and awakening of your third eye chakra.
- When finished, close your eyes. You may see the image of the flame in your mind's eye.
- Notice if there are other colors you see behind your closed eyes. These are your aura.

- When this image dissolves, open your eyes and repeat if desired.

EXPANSIVE HEART-OPENING MEDITATION

Ease into a peaceful night's sleep by returning to the wisdom of your heart center in this reposeful meditation.

- Lie comfortably on your bed with your head supported and propped on a pillow.

- Close your eyes.

- Place your hands on your heart center with the left hand covering the right hand. This symbolizes the divine feminine supporting the male, as the right side of the body is the male side and the left is the female.

- Greet the divine with gratitude and request support.

- Inhale and exhale three or more steady breaths into and out of your heart center.

- Visualize the life force within you. See the radiant colors of your heart space: light pink, golden shimmer, and soft, steady white, all swirling within your center.

- Witness and observe your feelings. What are you seeing, feeling, experiencing in this moment?

- State what you are grateful for. Bask in and savor this feeling of appreciation. Enjoy thankfulness.

- Affirm your desired emotions and experiences.

- Ask your heart and the divine for wisdom and guidance in your subconscious dreams.

EVENING AFFIRMATIONS SLEEP MEDITATION

Pairing your breath with the repetition of reciting—either silently or out loud—positive, soothing affirmations right before you go to sleep can be transformative, imprinting these ideas into your subconscious as you slumber.

- Set your intention(s) by focusing on an affirmation or mantra.

- Prepare the ambiance of your bedroom for sleep. A Himalayan salt night-light offers a subtle, calming presence with soft light and the helpful, healing benefits of the salt.

- Lie down on your bed.

- Close your eyes and place your hands alongside your body, palms facing either up for receptivity or down for grounding. You may also choose to place your hands on your lower belly to feel the inflation and deflation of your physical body as you breathe in and out.

- Take a few moments to quiet and still your mind by beginning to breathe slowly, gently, and deeply.

- Focus on each inhalation and exhalation and how it feels.

- If a thought or nagging to-do pops into your head, allow yourself to let it go and refocus on your breathing. As with yoga, a meditation practice is just that—practice. Don't beat yourself up over it.

- Once you've cleared your inner voices, redirect your attention to your affirmations or intentions.

- Focus on these thoughts, and reflect on them.

- As you inhale, use that as an opportunity to breathe new life into these intentions, filling your lungs with fresh air and your body, brain, and heart with the affirmation of your choosing.

- As you exhale, use that as an opportunity to expel old air, stagnant energy, or any doubt or tension.

- Repeat as desired until you feel relaxed completely and ready for rest.

Summary

Practice these mindful meditation exercises as a regular part of your pre-bedtime routine—or anytime you need a reset to relax. Making meditation a daily habit will vastly improve your response, physically and emotionally, to external stressors, allowing you to quiet the body and brain for a soothing night of healing sleep.

CHAPTER 6
THE POWER OF POSITIVE AFFIRMATIONS AND BELIEF

Awakening Our Inner Healing with Our Mind's Eye

"What you seek is seeking you."

—Rumi

How we speak to ourselves—along with how often and how repetitively—is powerful. The words we choose and the stories we tell ourselves deeply impact our internal psyche as well as the way we present ourselves and our energy into the external world.

Our minds are powerful forces. So too is the inner area of our mind's eye, our third eye chakra, behind which is where the pineal gland is located, deep within the brain. If we can learn to harness the power of what we believe, then we can take a positive belief that our pineal gland is performing at its optimum functionality and transform this healing thought into physically healing action. Because the pineal gland also plays a role in the production of serotonin, which generates a feeling of well-being, we can use this process to amplify our emotions and inner healing abilities.

The law of attraction explains that our minds and, therefore, our experiences, are like magnets: What you put out into the universe is what will magnetize back to you. For example, positive thoughts will attract more positive experiences into your life and negative thoughts magnetize similar negative experiences. Similarly, if you wake up believing you're feeling unwell, then it's likely that your body will manifest physical symptoms that correlate with those feelings. On the other side of the coin, if you wake up feeling well rested and grateful for a good night's sleep (thank you, high-functioning pineal gland and adequate melatonin levels!), then along with all the opportunities available to you over the coming day, you'll also be more open and receptive to allowing and receiving the flow of more good things to come.

Once a story becomes a part of you, any recollection of it will bring up the feeling that comes with that narrative. That being said, the constant chatter running through your brain (your narrative) influences the way you think and feel. Change this narrative and the way your brain processes, thinks, and receives information, and your life too will change.

Words are vibrations. Sending out what you want to channel can help activate your purpose and presence of mind. You can tap into the powerful energy of storytelling by speaking aloud to yourself each day, morning and night. Reciting in a repetitive nature words that convey transformative, positive affirmations can–and will–reprogram the nature of your thoughts and actions.

REFRAME YOUR NARRATIVE

As mentioned above, how we view and feel about the narratives that shape our lives is crucial in how our energy radiates—or how it detaches. Use the following prompts to shift and reframe your narrative into one that will positively influence your body, mind, and spirit.

⚹ How am I feeling about my energy and vibe today?

....

⚹ How can I change or reframe this feeling into one that feels better?

....

⚹ What can I say to give myself a pep talk?

....

⚹ How would feeling better alter the course of my day, how I feel physically within my body, and my emotional health?

....

- What, if anything, can I do to shift what I am feeling or experiencing?

....

- What else do I want to tell myself that is positive and helpful?

....

Immediately upon waking, make the very first words you speak to yourself—even before you get out of the calm, peaceful nature of your bed—ones of a positive nature. Equally as important: make expressions of gratitude an early priority as you move into your day. By cultivating an attitude of gratitude and positivity right off the bat, you recalibrate the brain, raising your energetic vibration and purposefully setting the tone with mindful intentions.

SHARING HEALING ENERGY

To send your healing energy out to others, try the following steps:

- Ground yourself in gratitude, breath, and self-awareness.
- Visualize an energetic connection between yourself and others. Through this connection, offer up an intention to help or heal.
- Set the intention to manifest by opening up your heart, feeling and expressing unconditional love.
- Have faith and trust in the universe that your energy has been received.

To expand upon affirmations and mantras, let's group them into times of day.

Morning Mantras

Initiate an early morning routine that trains your brain to begin each day from a place of abundance and love.

POSITIVE MORNING RITUAL

Try this ritual every morning. For an ongoing practice, make use of a separate notebook. Keep this book or the notebook on your nightstand so that you can easily access it without having to get up.

✎ Write the phrase "I AM GRATEFUL" and list at least three things you feel gratitude for.

✎ Next, write down the phrase "I AM MANIFESTING," "I AM INTENTIONAL," or "I AM DOING" and list the items you would like to integrate into your day.

✎ Recite the lists aloud.

EVENING AFFIRMATIONS

Perform these affirmations prior to bedtime in order to allow them to be fully absorbed into your subconscious as you sleep.

- ⚘ Write the phrase "Amazing Things That Happened Today" and list three (or more) of the day's activities or happenings that made you feel grateful. It just might make you smile to relive these events and their joyful emotions!

- ⚘ Write the phrase "I AM MANIFESTING" or "I AM INTENT ON" and beneath it list items you'd like to put into action.

- ⚘ Place this book on your nightstand or next to your pillow to harness the power of subconscious thought manifesting into action.
- ⚘ You can repeat the Positive Morning Ritual and the Evening Affirmations using the templates provided on page 120.

When using the power of positivity and intentional affirmations, words that convey positive actions (e.g., "I am running" or "I am doing a race") are a necessity. Conversely, words that have a connotation (e.g., "I am trying to run" or "I hope to do a race") can set us up for failure. It is key to focus on intentional words of affirmation as a method of transforming those thoughts into realities.

JOURNALING PROMPTS

When putting pen to paper, it can be helpful to ask ourselves questions to discover what we need to release and what we would like to invoke. Here are some prompts for setting intentions and affirming your thoughts so that they may transform into realities.

🪶 What brought me gratitude today? What could bring me gratitude in the future?

🪶 Who or what can me give support, and how? Where do I need support?

🪶 What is working and why? What is not working? How could letting go of attachments help my growth?

≋ What could I stop doing?

≋ What could I start doing?

≋ What are the feelings and emotions I desire to experience?

🖋 How can I be more open?

🖋 What are nourishing thoughts or words that I can return to?

🖋 How can I bring clarity to my intentions?

🖎 How can I feel and be more free?

🖎 What can I do to prioritize myself?

🖎 How can I offer self-care to myself?

🖎 How can I believe in myself more?

✍ Who or what is in my heart?

✍ How can I harness my loving energy?

Summary

Our energy, words, and emotions influence all areas of our physical and mental health. By stimulating the areas within our brains, such as the pineal gland, that tap into our inner healing capabilities, we can amplify the levels of important hormones like melatonin—the secret to healthy, healing sleep—and serotonin—the key to a happy, joyous, positive life.

CHAPTER 7
MANIFESTING WITH THE POWER OF THE MOON

Connecting with the Fluidity of the Tides

*"Just as the water reflects the stars and the moon,
the body reflects the mind and soul."*

—Rumi

The moon moves through its phases of crescent and gibbous every two weeks, and along with it, so should your energy. The moon is a vibrant force, the regulator of the ebb and flow of the tides. Like the ocean, our physical bodies are primarily water. The shape-shifting moon is your connection to a higher power. The lunar bond that links the physicality of our bodies with the spiritual and natural elements of the world we inhabit is magical. This connection can help us go beyond our rational minds to inhabit our true spiritual and divine selves.

Manifestation is a process of channeling energy and emotion into vibrations. It brings thoughts into form or physical action and the desires of your heart into actuality. These acts of manifestation require you to engage with a deeper density of matter, calling in energy to create a new form. In turn, this has the powerful effect of tethering energy to the earth. If you manifest from an ungrounded place, your manifestations will be fleeting and temporal. If you manifest from a place of rooting down and lifting up, then you can influence both the heart and the spirit, inhabiting a healthy, high-vibration, positive space of creation from both elements.

The new moon is a powerful time for manifesting, setting intentions, beginning new chapters, and tapping into fresh, empowering, receptive energy. Two weeks later comes the full moon, a time for letting go, releasing what no longer serves us, and making productive use of freeing, weightless energy.

With this framework in mind, we can harness the power of sacred rituals. Because the moon's light is more intense at night, practicing these sacred moon ceremonies in the evening hours can utilize the full power of the moon and moonlight. In turn, these celebratory rituals can help to activate and awaken the power of the mind in manifesting an opening of the third eye chakra to enhance our intuitive clarity.

After all, the sleeping hours are when our subconscious takes over—and often what appears in our dreams is a clarity of consciousness that our minds are unable to tap into while we are physically awake. This is where the importance of the pineal gland comes into play: the pineal gland creates the proper levels of melatonin to regularize our sleeping cycles, as well as the serotonin needed to bring our emotions to open fluidity. When these processes are working at their best, our third eye can awaken, activate, and be open to receive the intuition that comes from within our subconscious sleep state. These aspects can become even more powerful on the nights of a new or full moon.

When performing any ritual, including those related to the moon, it's best to move from the heart and its emotions. Doing something simple and heartfelt is far more effective and powerful than performing a pomp-and-circumstance ceremony that doesn't connect or resonate with your soul.

Intentionally selecting your focus during these ceremonies is essential. These curated thoughts will become realities, imprinted with the feelings, emotions, and intentions of what you are seeking to create. This will allow them to manifest into full fruition. Once you integrate this practice into your life, then your spirit, soul, and life will become alive.

NEW MOON

Perform these rituals when the moon is waxing—from the new moon to the peak of the full moon—to manifest new life chapters as well as to increase, enhance, or strengthen relationships. The new moon is a potent time of fresh energy, new beginnings, and connection with the power of creation.

FULL MOON

Full moon rituals, performed after the full moon's peak until just before it once again becomes a new moon (a period known as the waning moon), are best for banishing things that are unwanted or weighing us down. The full moon allows us to release stuck, stagnant energy, freeing us of ties that bind. This is a powerful time for transformation and change.

PERFORMING AN EFFECTIVE RITUAL

To bring your ritual to fullest fruition, consider these elements:

- Be extremely clear and detailed with your intentions.
- Choose an altar, vision board, or other creative outlet to reflect your intentions.
- Arrange reflective items (think: a mirrored tray or mirrored jewelry box) in a mindful manner. For example, a circular shape is symbolic of a consistent spiral of cyclical, positive energy, and a heart shape can symbolize pure love. These mirrored objects are also symbolic of the pure, reflective light of your heart's desires and intentions.
- Approach the higher power, divinity, or your spiritual guide and ask for help.
- Affirm and pray for the best and highest outcome for all beings.
- Be faithful, and trust that the ritual process will work.
- Remain focused in this attitude, confident that what you're seeking is already on its way.
- Practice and express gratitude continuously. The more thankful we are, the higher our vibration is, allowing energy to magnetize.
- Keep your heart open to the wisdom of the universe and its guidance.

NEW MOON RITUAL

Determine what the astrological sign is for this moon phase. This can help you set clear intentions that align with the astrology of the universe. When the moon is in this new moon phase, it's the place of planting the seeds of creation. Here, as in all types of conception, we can use this power to create new life.

- Treat yourself with self-care by practicing an activity that is meaningful for you, whether it's a salt bath, yoga routine, meditation, journaling, or a combination of all of these. Cleanse and unwind.

- Find a sacred space.

- Light a candle and, if desired, burn palo santo or sage.

- Arrange your crystals, altar, or vision board.

- Write down in ink—rather than pencil, which can be erased—what you wish to manifest in the coming days. Be as specific and detailed as possible. Putting pen to paper is a powerful practice.

- Then, hold these intentions close to your heart as you recite them out loud.

- Close your eyes and breathe life into these desires. Visualize the intentions as if they are already occurring, and feel the emotions of gratitude and joy.

- Place the paper, along with any crystals, directly in the light of the moon. This can be outdoors, if available, or on a windowsill. (See Chapter 8 for information on crystals.)

- If desired, fill a glass jar or pitcher with "moon water." To make moon water, fill a clear container of your choosing with filtered or distilled water. Place the vessel in the same spot as your crystals and handwritten intentions, directly under the moonlight. Use this charged moon water on subsequent days for cleansing or drinking in order to fully absorb the moon's power.

FULL MOON RITUAL

For full moon rituals, follow the same steps, but list out those things you want to release or let go of. Think of what is no longer serving you and write it down. You can burn this list to symbolize the act of letting go with ease and gratitude. Be sure to carry out any burning in a fire-safe, controlled setting with extinguishing tools on hand.

Summary

Try practicing both new and full moon ritual exercises in self-care. Include the elements discussed in this chapter or customize each practice to suit your unique desires and needs.

CHAPTER 8
MAKING MAGIC WITH HEALING CRYSTAL GEMSTONES

Energy Crystals to Elevate the Pineal Gland

"Walk as if you are kissing the earth with your feet."

—Thich Nhat Hanh

Because of my name—Crystal—I have always been intrigued by and interested in crystal gemstones. Crystal gemstones contain a fascinating well of healing energy. Magic happens when we come into direct contact with crystals. Whether we are holding one within our hands or wearing one as jewelry, the energy of the crystal fuses with our own energetic field and vibrates with it in concert.

When we hold a crystal in our hands, the connection also stimulates chemical activity in areas such as the pineal gland. Certain crystal gemstones can become electromagnetically charged when you hold them, sending a signal to the brain that can activate the pineal gland. For this reason, the crystals we will discuss are directly linked to the hormones the pineal gland produces—melatonin and serotonin—which produce the emotions of ease, calm, relaxation, happiness, and joy, as well as intuition and awareness. These specific crystal gemstones are directly related to both the pineal gland and its energetic counterpart, the third eye chakra.

You might be wondering how this is possible. Crystals are imbued with the essence of our planet, and within them reside the powerful vibrations and energy of the universe. In addition, their origin within the earth infuses them with a grounding element.

As with all matter and souls and beings on the earth, including you, each and every crystal holds within it a unique and otherworldly vibration of energy. This cosmic imprint can be felt, translated, and understood by certain receptive souls, often known as empaths.

Crystal gemstones help us seek the connections we crave, providing power, spiritual wisdom, protection, healing, and, perhaps most importantly, the transmutation of energy that our spiritual selves and the divinity of our souls both need and crave. Crystal gemstones are keepers of time and energy and record holders of wisdom, helping and guiding us to lead more meaningful, empowered, abundant, and intentional lives.

The number of known crystal types changes year by year. Most crystals are made up of various minerals, while minerals are materials in and of themselves. Every year, on average of thirty to fifty new minerals are identified, though not all are confirmed. According to the Mineralogical Society of America, there are approximately 4,000 identified and known minerals on the planet today.[5]

The third eye chakra is ruled by the moon, and its corresponding colors are shades of indigo blue bordering on blue-purple. Crystals commonly associated with this chakra include some of these blue gems:

- Apatite
- Aquamarine
- Blue aventurine
- Labradorite
- Lapis lazuli
- Tanzanite

Know Your Crystals

Chakra Crystal: Apatite

Apatite is a crystal reputed to be mystical in nature and valued for stimulating metaphysical abilities. It is also thought to be the gem that guides the metabolic system via the chakras. All apatite stimulates the pineal gland, famously described by the philosopher Descartes as "the seat of the soul." When we fully activate our pineal gland, we can experience "the spirit molecule," a secretion known as dimethyltryptamine, or DMT. This is a natural psychedelic involved in exceptional out-of-body experiences.

---

5.   Hobart M. King, "What Are Minerals?" accessed November 8, 2021, https://geology.com/minerals/what-is-a-mineral
.shtml#:~:text=There%20are%20approximately%204000%20different,%2C%20solubility%2C%20and%20many%20more.

Apatite is a crystal rich in calcium and hydroxyapatite, a mineral produced within the body and a major component of tooth enamel and bones, along with phosphorus. Hydroxyapatite is found in "brain sand," which consists of the calcified areas found in parts of the brain, including those that are present in the pineal gland. Calcification impairs the function of the pineal gland. As the pineal gland has also been known to monitor and regulate the effects of electromagnetic fields, in turn, this process of regulating/monitoring calcification makes it of utmost importance for the decalcification and optimum function of our third eye chakra.

Calcium imbalances can potentially be treated or healed harnessing the healing powers of the apatite crystal. An overaccumulation of fluorite, a form of fluoride, within the pineal gland has a negative and detrimental impact on our sleep patterns. Apatite can help the pineal gland dissolve these accumulations and reestablish balance as it energetically releases excess calcium and fluoride. Apatite may also help with hypertension that is caused by an overabundance of calcium in the body. Tap into this decalcifying healing by placing an apatite crystal over joints, bones, or directly on your third eye chakra. When held on your third eye, blue apatite will accelerate your rational mind in integrating and enhancing its intuitive abilities. Apatite is also thought to balance the hemispheres of the brain, stimulating neurotransmitters and tapping into both the right- and left-brain modes of perception.

Chakra Crystal: Aquamarine

The term "aquamarine" is connected with the color of the sea's blue waters. This ties in to the stone's use as a healing, calming crystal that lends itself to spiritual vision, allowing you to reach a higher state of awareness.

Use this crystal as a healing and harmonizing stone for imbalanced glands by holding it directly on your brow to sharpen and cultivate clear mental perception. Aquamarine is also powerful for harnessing hope and calming overactive minds.

Chakra Crystal: Blue Aventurine

Blue aventurine is a crystal linked to fertility of life and ideas, to expansion and growth. In fact, aventurine helps anything to grow—including you! All things—plants, your drive, your motivation—flourish and thrive in the presence of this crystal stone. It also brings good fortune and luck to new ventures. Your growth can occur internally, spiritually, or emotionally, allowing for your evolution to a higher state of consciousness, cosmic connection, and awareness.

This crystal is a versatile and healing stone, resonating energetically with the thymus gland and immune system. It facilitates inner calm and mental healing. Try infusing water with aventurine by adding the crystal to a glass, bottle, or dish filled with water. Blue aventurine is an excellent aura protector, guarding against electromagnetic emissions such as blue light.

Blue aventurine disconnects you from anything that is sapping your power. This is a stone of joyous abundance, helping you rebuild any lacking feelings and transform them into focused clarity of mind and openness to all the wondrous possibilities in life.

Chakra Crystal: Labradorite

As the primary crystal of the new moon, labradorite helps us to rely on our own intuition when we are lacking the moon's direction. Labradorite can accelerate our spiritual growth and development, assisting us in focusing our thoughts to create clarity in our intentions and deepest desires. It is also a stone that creates space for communication. As the blue and indigo hues align with your throat and your third eye chakra, you are able to open up and speak with wisdom from your heart. You can also use the many flashes of fire within this crystal as a focus for a gazing meditation.

Chakra Crystal: Lapis Lazuli

Lapis lazuli is known as the currency of queens and is representative of the night sky. This crystal symbolizes cosmic correspondence and the idea that what is visible below is a reflection of what exists above, carrying and sharing vibrations of energy, like the ocean reflecting the sky.

Use this stone, which stimulates the immune system, for healing diseases related to the eyes as well as for help in the process of detoxification. The crystal can also be used to access the blissful state of "heaven on earth" when incorporated into a meditation practice. Meditating with lapis lazuli stimulates the third eye chakra, allowing us to foster increased access to higher levels of conscious awareness. The crystal's high electrical conductivity channels purity of existence, transforming blockages—emotional or mental—to set your spirit free.

Chakra Crystal: Tanzanite and Tanzine Aura Quartz

Aura quartzes activate the spiritual and energetic body, grounding it in the physical body. When laid along the chakras like a rainbow, these quartz colors raise the vibrational rate of each chakra to allow for an expanded state of consciousness. Aura quartzes are a basis for spiritual alchemy and act as powerful tools for expansion and guidance of your soul and spirit. Tanzanite is a crystal that can help bring the body back into alignment, especially for those experiencing blockages due to excessive fluoridation. The crystal acts almost as a subtle antibiotic, eliminating pathogens both physical and metaphysical. This stone can also transmute negative emotions and help restore cellular function. Use these crystal stones to transform negative emotions into positive ones.

Three Other Third Eye Chakra Crystals: Apophyllite, Banded Agate, and Celestite

- An apophyllite crystal stone can be placed on your third eye chakra to create a calm mind, eradicate confusion, and enhance mental clarity.

- Place a banded agate crystal stone directly on your third eye chakra to remove any ties to an authority figure whom you have outgrown or evolved away from.

- Use a celestite crystal stone on your third eye chakra to open up the portal to psychic communication with the cosmic world of celestials.

DISCOVER WHICH CRYSTAL GEMSTONES YOU NEED RIGHT NOW

Use the following questions as a connectivity guide, then go back to the Know Your Crystals section to determine which crystal gemstone is right for you in this moment.

- What are my emotions and feelings right now?

- What do I wish to bring into my life?

✍ What do I need to release from my life?

✍ Does color, texture, or another element draw me to a particular crystal?

✍ What areas in my life need healing?

✍ What do I need to become more aware of?

✍ What do I wish to magnetize into my life?

✍ How clear are my thoughts?

- Do I need to trust myself and my intuition more?

- Am I feeling stuck or stagnant or blocked?

- Am I seeking creativity or inspiration?

- How can I increase my connection to myself and others?

- Does one of these crystal gemstones resonate with me or pull me toward it?

CLEANSING YOUR CRYSTALS

Upon receiving any new crystals into your space, it's imperative to cleanse them. This will erase any previous energy (consider others who may have held the stones, or ways they may have been transported to you) and allow a fresh state unique to you.

To cleanse crystals, there are a few options:

- Place the crystals in the soil of a healthy houseplant for twenty-four hours.
- Set the crystals outdoors under the light of the sun or a full moon for at least four hours.
- Immerse the crystals in the smoke of burning sage.
- Rinse the crystals in salt water, such as that of the ocean.

CHARGING YOUR CRYSTALS

You can charge your crystals under the light of a full or new moon.

- Set the crystals directly in moonlight, ideally outdoors on the soil of the earth (as opposed to in a pot).
- If outdoor space is unavailable, arrange the crystals in a bowl or on an altar of your choosing and place them on a windowsill that receives full or partial moonlight.

USING YOUR CRYSTALS FOR INTENTIONS

Follow these steps to use the crystals of your choice for intention setting:

- Identify your intention. Examples could be "I am open," "I am inspired," "I am love," or anything that compels you.
- Hold the crystals within your palms.
- State aloud or silently within your mind: "I activate these stones."
- Recite or write down your intention eleven times.

1. ....

2. ....

3. --

4. --

5. --

6. --

7. --

8. --

9. --

10. --

11. --

- Whenever you experience a sense of blockage, burnout, or restlessness, take your crystals with you as you move through your day. Crystals respond to engagement and stimulation.

- When the blockage subsides, you can place the crystals in a sacred space in your home. (We will explore the creation of sacred spaces in Chapter 13.)

Summary

Whether you're feeling blocked or burned out or simply need a boost, allow the crystal stones of your choosing to help awaken your inner inspiration and motivation. They will work with you to bring a sense of balance, shift your perspective, inspire you, strengthen you, and guide you to release blockages in order to access a receptive state. The stones described in this chapter are ideal for harnessing your pineal gland power for producing melatonin and serotonin while also helping you to awaken and feel inspired, and to activate the awareness, intuition, and clarity of your third eye chakra.

CHAPTER 9
INTENTION SETTING AND GRATITUDE PRACTICE

Ask, Believe, Receive

"Watch your thoughts; they become your words. Watch your words; they become your actions. Watch your actions, they become your habits. Watch your habits; they become your character. Watch your character; for it becomes your destiny."

—Lao Tzu

Setting intentions is a powerful practice. By establishing a clear picture of how you want your state of being to feel and exist in relation to your external environment, you can channel the energy needed to raise your own vibration, accomplish your goals, and act with mindful consciousness.

Creating clear intentions every day, preferably both in the morning and the evening, will help you in the practice of manifestation techniques. While we cannot control all of our circumstances, we can choose both how we feel and how we react to every situation. Practicing this regulation of your responses will yield great results in your emotional and physical well-being. Regulating our emotions can alter and influence how we respond to the circumstances surrounding and within our lives. When the pineal gland is releasing melatonin, for example, we may feel the sense of calm, ease, and relaxation needed to fall—and stay—asleep. And when the pineal gland secretes serotonin, our brains generate happiness and joy, emotions that help us feel strong, powerful, and capable of manifesting the desires of our hearts. We can help better regulate and promote these positive emotions of relaxation, peacefulness, and happiness by bringing to mind a joyful moment or image, thus invoking and setting the tone for the day or sleeping hours to follow.

The universe responds to your vibration. It's the law of attraction: If you begin each day with a positive attitude and conscious intentions, that high-vibration energy will help you manifest, magnetize, and attract like experiences throughout your day. Conversely, if you start the day weighed down and generating low-vibration energy, waking up on the wrong side of the bed as they say, you're likely to experience a day filled with more of that energy.

Beginning the day with positive energy and loving emotions can propel our attitude and prep our energy for the coming twenty-four hours. When we connect with our heart's wisdom and emotional intelligence, we can move through the day and set higher intentions with depth and purpose. Use the following steps to complete a morning-to-evening checklist of wellness habits.

MORNING WELLNESS CHECKLIST

First things first. Before even getting out of bed, express gratitude and mindful intention. I like to speak aloud a positive and intentional affirmation immediately upon waking.

Next, establish your intentions and set a gratitude list for the day. Keep this book or another notebook on your nightstand. I believe in the power of putting pen to paper, which I follow with reciting the statements, speaking them aloud. Ink is important for establishing clear and permanent intentions. I use a red pen because red indicates the power of manifestation.

Choose at least three intentions and three things you are grateful for and write them down. These intentions should reflect your core desired feelings and preferred state of being, using phrases that embody high-vibration emotions. Think of phrases such as "I am," "I receive," or "I give thanks for" and use these as guidelines to set the tone for your day.

Select nourishing thoughts that encourage and generate positive feelings. Make an intention to generate actions that help you, and the world, experience the greatest good. Recognize that gratitude is a building block of abundance. As you make your gratitude list, describe in detail why you are grateful for each item. Be specific. This will increase thankfulness and generate further waves of gratitude.

Weekly and Monthly Intention Setting

Take the time at the beginning of each week and month to sit down and write by hand a list of what you wish to experience in that time. Forming and creating such a list is the ultimate act of both self-care and manifesting potential!

INTENTION SETTING

- ꙮ Find a space of stillness and quiet.

- ꙮ Gather your notebook and planner, some colored pens, and a mug of your favorite healing elixir, tea, or coffee.

- ꙮ Plan your opening ritual by creating a visioning page or pages. Create your own visioning page in the blank space on page 84.

THE HEALING POWER OF THE PINEAL GLAND

✎ Write down a gratitude list.

✎ Write down your intentions, as well as the actionable steps you will take to make them manifest.

✎ Define your priorities for the coming days.

- -

- -

- -

- -

- -

Making Mantras

Creating and setting mantras or core focus ideations for the days to come in the week or month ahead is also helpful.

MAKING A MANTRA LIST

Create a mantra list with affirmative phrases like those below. Keep the list in a visible location.

- What is meant for me will find me.
- I allow what is meant for me to come into my life.
- I have faith in the universe.
- I trust in the timing and pace of my life.
- I trust that all is going according to divine order.
- I am open and receptive to what flows to me.
- Expect miracles and they will manifest.
- Radiate positive energy.
- Choose joy.
- Energy flows where my intentions go.

- Be thankful.
- Share and express love.

(blank lined writing space)

Summary

Creating clearly defined intentions infused with positive energy will help raise the vibrations of your state of being. Tap into the power of gratitude, intention setting, and regulating your emotional responses to build better daily habits.

CHAPTER 10
BRAIN DETOX JOURNALING

Write It Down and Release It

"The thinking mind is what is busy. You have to stay in your heart. You have to be in your heart. Be in your heart. The rest is up here in your head where you are doing, doing, doing."

—Ram Dass

Prioritizing self-care is not selfish. Rather, it's a key part of internal regulation, both emotionally and physically, as well as a factor in how we show up in the world. Without proper self-care, we do not have the tools to return to our center, our clarity, or our faith, nor do we have the capacity or energy to be of service to others. As the saying goes, "You can't pour from an empty cup."

If stress, anxieties, worries, tasks, or other lingering thoughts or nagging to-do's are cluttering your mind, this can hamper the pineal gland's performance. Learning how to let go, release, and clear out the clutter can prepare the pineal gland to complete its responsibilities: producing the melatonin and serotonin needed for you to release, relax, reset, restore, rejuvenate, and recalibrate at bedtime and overnight as you sleep.

Both professionally and personally, I prioritize making the most of my mornings and evenings by practicing self-care routines. These routines optimize the physical health and emotional wellness of the most important person in my life: myself. Scheduling time for self-care results in spiritual growth and can help us expand our relationship with ourselves as well as with those around us.

For me, and perhaps for you as well, journaling before bed relaxes my mind for an optimum night of sleep. I call my pre-sleep journaling routine a "brain dump" or "brain detox." In other words, this is the time to jot down every single thought, to-do, or other item that pops into your mind.

By transferring this list of swirling thoughts to paper, we can get it out of our heads. This acts as a detoxification, releasing thoughts from binding us and keeping us up at night.

This evening activity allows you to free your mind of pesky inner voices and nagging thoughts of undone tasks that pop up when you're trying to fall asleep, or worse yet, wake you up at 3:00 a.m. before an important morning meeting.

PRE-BEDTIME BRAIN-DUMP JOURNALING

Settle into your bed for this therapeutic activity. Getting those endless to-do's out of your head and onto a piece of paper is cathartic.

- Write down the date and time. This way, you can refer to the list later to see which actions have aligned with your intentions.

Date: _____ Time: _____

- Spend the next several minutes free-writing whatever flows into your mind. Don't edit or censor.

🖎 When you're finished, close this book and put it away, out of your direct line of vision. Out of sight, out of mind!

Summary

Make those few precious moments before bed count for a daily self-care practice. Integrate a journaling habit into your nightly routine. Use the time before sleep as a practice in releasing any troublesome or nagging thoughts onto paper. This way, your brain can sleep easy without worrying about your internal checklist.

CHAPTER 11
ELEVATED EVENING AFFIRMATIONS

Invoking Visualization to Manifest in Your Dreams

"The next message you need is always right where you are."

—Ram Dass

As with morning intentions, how we end our day is of great importance—especially for the levels of melatonin that regulate our sleep. It is important for your pineal gland, along with the rest of your mind and body, to take time before sleep to disconnect from the events of the day. This will allow you to reset your system and create the calm state and flow of melatonin that are necessary for a good night's sleep.

You might want to try a soothing, restorative yoga sequence from Chapter 3, read a book, use the journaling prompts below, or enjoy a cup of tea—whatever helps you turn off your running to-do list and transition your brain to a relaxed state. This also allows your pineal gland to work efficiently in creating those hormones that act as a catalyst for improved sleep and healthier rest.

JOURNALING PROMPTS

✎ What thoughts and actions can I take to help me feel the way I want to feel?

....

....

☞ What are my key beliefs?

☞ What positive statements can give me comfort and guide me in my subconscious state of sleep?

EVENING AWARENESS AFFIRMATIONS

☞ What do I want to ruminate on?

☞ What intentional actions do I want to take tomorrow?

☞ What do I want to manifest tomorrow?

🕊 How can my actions tomorrow be of good to me and of service to others?

🕊 What are my three priorities for tomorrow?

🕊 What are three things I am grateful for this evening?

You may wish to keep this page open on your nightstand or next to your pillow so the intentions can drift into your subconscious as you sleep.

"You are what your deep, driving desire is. As your desire is, so is your will. As your will is, so is your deed. As your deed is, so is your destiny."

—Brihadaranyaka Upanishad

One of the most ancient Vedic texts, the Upanishads are one of the foundations of Hinduism. The quotation above is a personal favorite—it emphasizes and articulates the power of our minds. Once we have painted a clear picture of how we want, and more importantly, expect, things to go, we can make sure that our will manifests it into actuality.

Visualization is a practice that helps us manifest our dreams into existence. By holding images of the experiences we wish to manifest, as well as feeling the corresponding emotions as if the experiences were actually happening, we can channel this energy into invoking these events into reality.

This exercise will help you retrieve and receive wisdom from your consciousness and become inspired by the magic of life. Practicing visualization, both right before going to sleep and first thing upon waking in the morning, will help manifest what you want into your life.

VISUALIZATION-INVOKING EXERCISE

- Sit in a comfortable space where you will not be disturbed.

- Close your eyes, breathe deeply, and imagine what you are seeking to welcome into your life.

- As you visualize, try to fully experience each sensation, emotion, and feeling that the experience will bring to you.

- Hold these feelings as if the event were happening in the present moment.

By creating the image along with feeling its elements, you can tap into your pineal gland, your third eye chakra, and your brain's power to transform these mental images into actualized reality.

Summary

The practices covered in this chapter may also help with the detoxification of the pineal gland so that it can effectively produce melatonin and serotonin. While the pineal gland is self-regulating, it can still fall prey to inactivity, disruption, disability, or suppression. These exercises are examples of how to give the pineal gland a boost.

Visualization invoking can be a powerful process for facilitating the path to lucid dreaming, in which we are conscious that we are, in fact, dreaming, which is directly linked to the function of the pineal gland. You can improve lucid dreaming by giving melatonin levels a boost; the higher the levels of melatonin, the higher the quality of your dreams during the night. Lucid dreaming can also be a result of earlier visualization techniques, allowing your third eye chakra to be fully open during your subconscious state and increase the quality of your dreams. You may awaken the next day with newfound clarity and awareness!

CHAPTER 12
LYMPHATIC DRAINAGE AND MINDFUL MOVEMENT

Stimulating Circulation and Detoxing the Body for Better Rest

"You cannot always control what goes on outside. But you can always control what goes on inside."

—Wayne Dyer

I find that both my brain and my body work best when I make movement a must in my daily routine, ideally first thing in the morning.

Whether it's yoga, Pilates, bicycling, or a walk, making movement a morning priority can be extremely helpful in setting the tone for your day. Checking off this important item first thing can boost both your mental and physical states. And if your workout is done in the morning, later excuses can't derail you from getting that daily dose of endorphin-elevating exercise!

Research shows that regular movement and exercise alleviate stress, so get those endorphins flowing and your blood circulation pumping. Exercise and movement also create clarity of mind, which helps us focus and concentrate throughout the day. The physical and mental health boost from movement will energize, sooth, and stabilize your system, leading to a better night's sleep.

Lymphatic drainage is a useful tool for releasing stagnant energy. Releasing congestion that has manifested within our physical bodies allows our minds, chakras, energy, nervous system, and glands to all work more efficiently. The pineal gland needs to produce both serotonin and melatonin effectively so the rest of the body's systems run smoothly. When systems are backed up or stuck, this cannot happen in an effective manner. Manual lymphatic drainage and mindful movement can help catalyze these actions.

Lymphatic drainage offers some of these emotional and physical health benefits:

- Improved immune function and support
- Increased blood circulation and tissue regeneration
- Promotion of lymphatic flow for quicker elimination of excess fluid
- Reduced swelling, puffiness, and water retention
- Elimination of toxins
- Soothing of body and mind
- Enhanced feeling of lightness in the body
- Mental clarity

Lymphatic fluid is a clear liquid that circulates throughout the body, acting as a method of elimination to facilitate your natural detoxification process. Lymphatic fluid works to cleanse and flush the arteries and connective tissues. The lymphatic system does not have a pump to push lymphatic fluid around the body the way the heart moves blood. Because of this, lymphatic fluid relies mainly on the muscle action of the body to stimulate movement. Enter manual lymphatic drainage massage.

This massage technique can be performed by a professional or at home using a lymphatic drainage massage tool such as a paddle. The massage process stimulates the movement of lymphatic fluid toward the lymph nodes, which are located mainly in the armpits, neck, and groin area. The aim is to accelerate the removal of excessive fluid, directing it toward the capillary vessels using specific movements to effectively eliminate it.

DIY LYMPHATIC DRAINAGE MASSAGE

To perform your own lymphatic drainage massage, try the following routine:

- Gather a wooden lymphatic massage paddle and a moisturizing oil.

- Rub the oil into the areas you will be massaging. This step is important for protecting the skin as you manipulate it with the paddle.

- Begin by awakening your lymphatic system by pumping the major lymph nodes.

Pump the back of the knees and the armpits five times each.

- Next, holding the paddle in a horizontal position, start stroking gently, moving from the ankle toward the inner thigh. Do three to seven strokes per leg.

- Then, flip the paddle to a vertical position and gently move from the ankle up the outer thigh. Repeat three to seven times per leg.

- Now, massage the back of the legs using the paddle held again in a vertical position. You can prop up your legs on a chair to allow for easier access behind the knees. Move in an upward motion until you hit the gluteal fold between your upper thigh and buttock.

- Finally, massage your arms with the paddle held in a vertical position. Move from wrist to armpit; repeat on the outer arm. Do three to seven strokes per arm.

FACIAL LYMPHATIC DRAINAGE

To drain lymph from the face, use this routine:

- Choose a skin care serum and mix it with a drop or two of facial oil.

- Dab or rub the serum on to your face, forehead, and neck in a downward motion.

- You can also use a rose quartz or jade gua sha tool, a stone massage tool or facial roller, to help the serum deeply penetrate the skin and increase the lymphatic drainage.

- Using the crystal tool of your choosing, start at the sinus points on the bridge of your nose.

- Pull gently with the tool to the side, then make a slight U shape and drag it downward. Do this three to five times.

- Then, move to the side of the jaw, using a similar action of sliding to the side and then dragging the skin—and with it, the lymphatic fluid inside—downward.

- Next, flip the tool (if using a gua sha stone) to use the flat edge under the chin, stroking down the neck into the collarbone. This is a key step in moving the fluid to drain downward toward the heart.

- Finally, if desired, you can smooth any fine lines in the forehead by gently stroking your brow in an upward motion.

Summary

Make movement and the healing power of touch a daily priority. From soul to spirit to mind to body, utilizing massage and movement practices can help alleviate and release stagnant energy, unblock resistance, and release physical tightness or stress. Integrate these mindful practices to your routine to elevate your emotional, physical, and energetic wellness.

CHAPTER 13
SETTING UP AND STYLING YOUR BEDROOM AS A SACRED SPACE FOR SLEEP

Rest with Ease in a Serene Sleep Space

"You are what you want to become."

—Thich Nhat Hanh

Your home is an extension of your energy. Because your physical space is reflective of your energetic being, how you set up this space is important. Think of this as a physical exercise in arrangement in order to cultivate what you want to manifest into your life.

If you're surrounded by clutter, it's likely that your mind will feel the same, and your thoughts may be scattered and unclear. The good news is that the opposite is also true: if your home, and specifically your bedroom, is organized, intentionally arranged, free of clutter, and peaceful, it's likely that you'll be able to relax and breathe easily. The calm, soothing sanctuary of your bedroom will become a place you'll look forward to settling into for a reset through a healthy night's sleep.

Because our mind can mirror our physical space, creating a sanctuary in your bedroom that exudes ease and calm is a key element in achieving better sleep. To ensure that the pineal gland works efficiently and effectively, take a survey of your bed and bedroom space. Does the area make you feel calm, relaxed, and at ease? If so, great; your pineal gland is probably producing serotonin followed by melatonin as we speak! If not, it may be time to do a deep clean and revamp your bedroom's surroundings, bedding, or even your bed itself. Let's begin!

For optimal sleep, the ideal environment will promote positivity, relaxation, and calm. Refreshing this intimate, sacred space—one where you spend approximately a third of your life—has the power to reframe your perspective on comfort, security, safety, and stability. Aside from the physical benefits of sleep, recalibrating your mind has the capability to help you rechannel any swirling or chaotic energy into a calmer state that is ready for rest.

Change is often a transformative catalyst for action. On the other hand, resistance or refusal to change can lead to stagnation and inaction. Even the smallest, simplest change to your everyday routine—at bedtime and elsewhere—can yield major results. So imagine how making changes on a large, broad scale can impact your quality of life and sleep!

First, the obvious: your bed. Upgrading your mattress and bedding (or better yet, both) can improve both the quantity and quality of your sleep. If you find yourself waking up every morning tired, despite how much sleep you've gotten, or with stiff, achy joints and a less-than-perky outlook, this may be a cue that it's time for a bedroom refresh.

Set Yourself Up for Sleep Success

Let's start with your mattress. In sleep as in any other physical activity, our bodies respond to the environment we are in as well as to the gear that is supporting us. You wouldn't run a marathon or go on a hike without being properly geared up, would you? Finding a mattress that properly supports your whole body is just as important.

Searching for the mattress that's "the one" is akin to the quest for the perfect partner. When seeking the right match, you flirt with a roster of options. At first glance, you're drawn to that fresh packaging, intrigued by its promises of potential. But your ultimate goal is a mattress that works for and supports your needs, growth, and wellness.

Much like finding a partner in life, starting with a checklist of needs and wants is helpful in selecting a mattress. I upgraded my mattress to a Stearns & Foster Luxury queen—and ever since then I look forward to going to bed and waking up well-rested in what I call "the cloud throne" because of its incredible softness and raised platform height. Here are things to consider and questions to ask yourself when choosing a mattress to support your bedtime habits and your body's unique needs.

SELECTING YOUR PERFECT MATTRESS

Consider these points when choosing a mattress to support your bedtime habits and your body's unique needs:

- First, think about how high off the ground you would prefer to sleep. This will help you to determine the depth of your mattress.

- Second, think about your sleeping positioning, bedding preferences, temperature preferences, and other habits. Also take into consideration whether it's likely to be just you in the bed or if you anticipate sharing the bed with a partner.

- Are you a side, back, or stomach sleeper?

- Do you prefer to sleep on a mattress that is soft, firm, or a combination of the two?

Better Bedding and Pillows

Your bedroom and your bed itself should be a sanctuary reserved for the three Rs: relaxation, romance, and rest. Consider upgrading your bedding and pillows to sumptuous materials that both feel luxurious and nourish your body and its needs.

Getting enough rest and establishing a healthy sleep cycle is dependent on many factors, including your body temperature. Your bedroom's temperature can have a significant impact on your sleep quality. According to a poll conducted by the National Sleep Foundation, a cool room temperature is one of the most important factors in getting a good night's sleep. The organization's findings were that the best bedroom temperature for a quality night of sleep is approximately 65°F (18.3°C).[6]

While this may vary by a few degrees from person to person, keeping the thermostat between 60–67°F (15.6–19.4°C) is optimum for the best night's sleep. With this in mind, switching up your sheets, pillowcases, and duvet to materials that promote coolness may be useful for maintaining a consistent, cool body temperature throughout the night. Breathable, moisture-wicking materials such as cotton, linen, silk, or satin can help promote better sleep. As an added bonus, these materials may help with allergies and respiratory health as well as being gentle on skin and hair.

6. Danielle Pacheco, "The Best Temperature for Sleep," June 24, 2021, https://www.sleepfoundation.org/bedroom-environment /best-temperature-for-sleep.

And not all pillows are created equal. It may be worth making the investment in a custom-crafted pillow such as the Pluto, which is built to your body's specifications and preferences and how you sleep. When picking a pillow, it's also essential to consider your sleeping position. For example, those with sleep apnea, acid reflux, allergies, or respiratory issues may find benefit from a higher pillow that can provide a slight angle to help promote drainage to alleviate overnight congestion.

Bedroom Feng Shui, Your Way

Establish your bedroom as your sacred sanctuary by creating harmony and balance using the principles of feng shui. Translated from the Chinese words for "wind" and "water," feng shui is believed to have been derived from an ancient poem describing human life as connected to and flowing with the surrounding environment.

This philosophy incorporates the practice of arranging the physical items in a space to create balance with the natural world. The goal is to harness energetic forces, establishing harmony between you and your environment. In this case, that environment is your bedroom and your bed itself.

We want to banish all mental and emotional intrusions from the bedroom, especially from the area directly surrounding the bed. No work, no screens (blue light from digital devices can disrupt our natural circadian rhythm and the brain's ability to fall asleep). And declutter, declutter, declutter!

Given that we spend eight or more hours each day in sacred space, elevating the energetic elements of feng shui principles in the bedroom areas surrounding your sacred place of rest may be beneficial in creating the needed clarity and spaciousness for both body and mind to unwind completely for a healthy night's sleep.

To put feng shui into practice, let's break down the basics.

- The commanding position: the focal point: This should be the primary space, the bed, where you spend the majority of the time while in the bedroom. This commanding position should be in a place farthest from the door or entry point and, ideally, diagonal to it, with a clear line of sight rather than directly in line with it. In turn, this balances the energy without placing your bed in a space where energy can be potentially channeled chaotically from entry and retreat.

- The bagua: the map that lets us evaluate the environment's energy field: This is a Chinese word that translates to "eight areas" that correlate to different life situations, such as career, family, or wealth. At the center of this area is a ninth area, which represents you and your overall wellness.

☞ The five elements: earth, fire, metal, water, wood: The five elements are phases in life that are interrelated and work together to connect and create a whole, complete system. Feng shui principles keep these five elements balanced both in your home space and within your life.

FENG SHUI YOUR BEDROOM

Now that we've outlined the basics, let's look at a checklist for how to apply feng shui to your bedroom.

☞ Begin by burning sage, palo santo, or cedar to clear the energy within the room. The aim is to banish any lingering, stuck, or stagnant energy from the space.

☞ Make sure the bed, the most important piece of furniture in this space, is in the focal point, or commanding position.

☞ Place the bed so it has diagonal sight access to the door without being directly in line with the door. This creates a sense of security and stability while avoiding threat.

☞ Do not position the bed directly underneath windows. Again, this fosters security and safety.

☞ Put up a headboard. Ideally, the headboard should be right up against the wall with ample room on either side for bedside tables. Headboards provide further feeling of support.

☞ Place a nightstand or side table on each side of the bed. This symbolizes the harmonious, loving energy of a pair. You can also use two similar or matching lamps on each end table and at least two pillows on the bed itself.

☞ Place plants (a minimal number; don't go overboard) strategically in the room. Snake plants and peace lilies are good options for purifying the air while you sleep, as they release high amounts of oxygen during the evening hours.

☞ Enhance the calm energy of your bedroom by keeping it free of electronic devices, heavy items, and items with sharp edges.

Bedroom Feng Shui Dos and Don'ts

DO make use of key colors. In feng shui, certain colors promote peacefulness, calm, relaxation, and sleep that is both productive and restful. Muted shades that you might find in nature, along with whites and creams, can be conducive to rest.

DO incorporate smell. Make use of essential oils, via a diffuser or candles. Lavender, jasmine, sandalwood, and eucalyptus are among the scents that promote healing, restful energy. We will explore more about scents in Chapter 14.

DO keep a glass of lemon-infused water on your nightstand to rehydrate and detoxify during the night.

DON'T use mirrors. A mirror in front of the bed can invite extra energy, disrupting the boundaries of your sleep space. Mirrors also reflect energy around your space, which can disrupt sleep.

DON'T use paintings or large photographs. These images can bring heavy or threatening energy.

DON'T keep clutter under the bed. The disorder can promote stress and chaotic energy.

Summary

Make the most of your bedroom by creating a peaceful, soothing vibe. Eliminate clutter and its corresponding energy. Make maintaining your bedroom space a practice in mindful minimalism. Select your bedding and colors with consciousness and keep the bedroom a place that promotes relaxation, healing, and more efficient sleep.

CHAPTER 14
HERBAL MAGIC IN ESSENTIAL OILS

How to Use Nature's Medicine for Soothing Sleep

"Set your life on fire. Seek those who fan your flames."

—Rumi

Scent has the powerful ability to correlate with significant experiences and instantly evoke strong memories and the feelings associated with remembered events.

This strong correlation arises from our sense of smell's direct connection to the brain and its centers of memory and emotion. Cells in the nose detect smells and send the information directly to the brain via the olfactory nerve. This then signals the limbic systems of the brain, including the amygdala, which control our memory and our emotional reactions. A whiff of something from the beach can trigger a calming vibe similar to the restful state created by melatonin. Or a waft of a fragrance connected to a happy memory can bring on an elevated emotion like one induced by a dose of serotonin from the pineal gland.

Smell is the only sense that moves directly to the brain's centers of emotion and memory instead of going to the relay station of the thalamus as other sensory information does.[7]

Here's where healing modalities such as aromatherapy and essential oils come into play. The ancient Greek physician Hippocrates studied essential oils and their effects and was a proponent of their healing, health-promoting properties.

Essential oils are believed to have a multitude of benefits, including promoting healthy sleep habits, relieving or reducing stress, alleviating pain, and regulating our mood. These oils have long been used to enhance relaxation and improve physical wellness. Essential oils may provide

7.   Marta Zaraska, *Discover Magazine*, "The Sense of Smell in Humans Is More Powerful Than We Think," October 10, 2017, https://www.discovermagazine.com/mind/the-sense-of-smell-in-humans-is-more-powerful-than-we-think.

relief from disruptive sleep patterns and improve sleep quality. The effects of essential oils may be compared to those of acupressure and massage. Using essential oils designed to promote sleep can improve both your sleep quality and your overall quality of life.

All the Essentials: Oils to Manifest Your Best Sleep Yet

In order to manifest your best sleep yet, make bedtime a total sensorial experience, utilizing the power of essential oils and scents as part of your routine. Here are some of the essential oils I recommend for improving the quality and quantity of your sleep:

Lavender: This is one the most well-known and popular essential oils for sleep and relaxation. Lavender has a soothing scent and has long been used as a natural remedy for anxiety. It has sedative effects and improves sleep quality, increases sleep quantity, and elevates a state of calm.

Vanilla: The sweet scent of vanilla has long been used for relaxation and stress relief. Vanilla can have a sedative effect, reduce hyperactivity and restlessness, calm and quiet the nervous system, relieve anxiety and depression, and lift your mood.

Rose and geranium: These two essential oils have similar floral scents. Both have been shown to reduce stress and anxiety, on their own and in combination with other essential oils.

Jasmine: Sweet and floral, jasmine is thought to improve sleep quality and reduce restlessness, all while alleviating anxiety and stress.

Sandalwood: Historically used for relaxation and anxiety relief, sandalwood has sedative effects that help to reduce alertness and wakefulness while promoting increased amounts of sleep.

Valerian root: Often referred to as nature's medicine, this herb is one of the plant kingdom's powerhouses. Filled with isovaleric acid, valerenic acid, and many antioxidants, valerian root has compounds that promote sleep, reduce anxiety, and break down aminobutyric acid, a chemical messenger that helps regulate nerve impulses in the brain and nervous system. By doing so, valerian root helps to create the same sort of calm and tranquility sometimes provided by prescription medications.

Chamomile: The calming effects of chamomile come from its wealth of the antioxidant apigenin. This molecule helps to reduce anxiety and stress, initiating the calm needed for sleep.

UTILIZING ESSENTIALS OILS FOR RELAXATION AND BETTER SLEEP

The following activities use scent and essential oils for sleep and relaxation:

- Take a bath. Using essential oils in a healing, soothing, end-of-day bath is a great antidote to any stressors. Soak in warm water infused with three to fifteen drops of essentials oils and Epsom salts approximately ninety minutes before bedtime to unwind, soak, and wash away the stressors of the day.

- Use an oil diffuser. Fill a diffuser with the oil of your choosing. The diffuser will disperse the essential oils throughout the air, increasing the state of calm, relaxation, and readiness for sleep.

- Create your own essential oil mist. You can combine an essential oil and water in a spray bottle, roll-on bottle, or atomizer. Mist your bedroom, bed linens, or body. To avoid irritation or other adverse reaction, use only four to five drops of oil for every half cup of water.

- Apply essential oil diluted with water to pressure points, such as on the wrists or behind the ears.

Keep in mind: Essential oils in undiluted form are highly concentrated and can irritate your skin. Do not apply an essential oil directly to the skin unless diluted with a barrier oil such as coconut oil.

Summary

Make the most of nature's medicine—plants— by infusing essential oils into your space or using aromatherapy with topical, roll-on essential oils. Allow their healing scents to remind you to take a moment, or several, to breathe, enjoy, and relax.

CHAPTER 15
TRAVEL AND GETTING GROUNDED IN NATURE

The Earth Element's Impact

"Travel brings power and love back into your life."

—Rumi

The better you feel, the more you allow. Allowing comes from a place of feeling your best and being receptive to the world's possibilities. This is where, why, and how the power of travel can shift our perspective and energy into that place of allowing, receptivity, and openness. Travel energizes our spirit, stirs our sense of wonder, and triggers new reactions in our brain.

How we dress and present ourselves to the world can do a great deal for our mental health. The terms "dopamine dressing" and "dressing for happiness" as described by the Brazilian brand Farm Rio explore the phenomenon of wearing certain colors, patterns, and prints to evoke positive emotions (think: the happy, relaxed beach vibe of a trip to Rio de Janiero). As with scent memory, dressing as if we are on a trip, for example, can make us feel the same uplifted emotions of being on vacation, even if we physically can't travel to a tropical island or commune with nature up in the mountains.

If we are fortunate enough to travel, it can boost our emotional and physical health, including that of our sleep cycle. Travel allows us to fully embrace all five of our senses while activating our pineal gland and third eye chakra with a sense of clarity and awakening.

Channeling that sense of energy from travel can lead to a boost in mental health, creativity, and purpose. Travel shows us life from a different perspective, presenting the potential and possibility of restructuring our own lives. Travel is the ultimate act of self care, one that allows us to go beyond our comfort zone and experience life in new ways.

What if you can't physically travel? Try a virtual vacation to one of your favorite destination or somewhere new by looking at photos or taking an online tour. Or, opt for a staycation or even a daycation near your own home or in your favorite nearby metropolitan area. Getting out of your daily routine and experiencing something new can tap into the creative potential of the mind and refresh any energy that feels stuck. You can even plan a vacation that might not manifest in physical form by visualizing yourself in the destination, feeling as if you are experiencing the emotions and sights of the place, without the hotel and flight costs. The anticipatory excitement and joy of planning travel is often as significant as the mental health benefits of actually taking the trip.

Nature and the power of "grounding" or "earthing"" are other facets of travel that can improve both our mental and physical health. Some studies suggest that spending time in the outdoors may improve your sleep. Camping, for example, can reset the body's alignment with nature's cycles of light and dark, which can result in longer, deeper, more productive sleep. The concept of grounding, or direct connection to the earth, is also helpful in balancing, nourishing, and reestablishing healthy sleep patterns.

Think of the earth as an enormous magnet containing reservoirs of energy, including energy found only within the ground. Everything—every object, every creature, every person—is connected with this electric force, and when we are grounded, we can tap into the interconnectedness that unites all entities across the universe.

More literally, being grounded means you are aligned, centered, balanced, stable, and strong, with minimal to no tension or stress. You are in union with your presence as a living being on this planet; your cells are connected and conducive to both emitting and receiving frequencies across your own system—muscular, skeletal, and nervous—as they are open to transmitting energy from other entities and the environment. As with all living beings on this planet, we are connected to the electric energy of the earth. In most societies, however, humans rarely go barefoot anymore, interfering with our ability to absorb this energy in the way many animals do. Shoes act as a barrier to the earth's energy; all the more so if you live or work in an urban environment or high-rise building.

There are many healing benefits linked to the practice of grounding. Some research has revealed that electrically conductive contact between the human body and the surface of the earth produces intriguing effects on the physiology and health of our bodies and brains. The effects may include these benefits:[8]

---

8. James Oschman et al., "The Effects of Grounding (Earthing) on Inflammation, the Immune Response, Wound Healing, and Prevention and Treatment of Chronic Inflammatory and Autoimmune Diseases," *Journal of Inflammation Research* 8 (March 24,

- Reduced stress

- Decreased inflammation and related pain

- Improved circulation

- Improved cell repair and function

- Proactive immune responses and wound healing

- Improvement in waste elimination and detoxification

- Restoration of homeostasis

- Mental calm

- Balance and stabilization

- Potential prevention and treatment of chronic inflammatory and autoimmune diseases

NATURAL WONDER: GROUNDING WITH THE EARTH EXERCISE

It's likely that you can't forgo wearing shoes altogether, but you can break the pattern of disconnection. The good news: going barefoot for even just half an hour has the potential to make a difference.

- First things first: ditch your shoes and any socks.

- Head outdoors.

- Sit, stand, or better yet, walk on the grass, sand, soil, or even concrete. From these conductive surfaces, your body can tap into the earth's healing energy.

- If possible, make this contact part of your daily routine to fully harness the healing power of the earth's energy. This energy will become intertwined with your own electromagnetic field, traveling through your internal energy field and all of your chakras, including that of your third eye chakra.

2015): 83–96, https://www.ncbi.nlm.nih.gov/pmc/articles/PMC4378297/.

Washing Away Worries: Ocean Healing for Mind, Body, and Soul

"I know of a cure for everything: salt water .... sweat, or tears, or the salt sea."

—Isak Dinesen

I am a self-proclaimed beach person and believe that anything that ails me—physical or emotional—can and will be helped by a trip to the shore. From the fresh, coastal breeze and roaring waves to awe-inspiring sunrises and sunsets and panoramic, never-ending horizons, observing the power of the tides brings restoration and reverence.

The beach and its horizon of the sky meeting the sea, with the waves crashing on the shore, are a moving meditation in and of themselves. This natural place of meditative reflection is one of the many reasons for the psychological link between the ocean and a state of calm contentment. And because the third eye chakra is linked with shades of aquamarine and other blue tones, being surrounded by these hues can help us to tap into the ocean's healing energy. The third eye chakra is also associated with light, and absorbing the beach's bright sun, whether we are sitting in stillness or walking on the sand, can help us to balance and open up this chakra.

The ocean's healing power is also homeopathically rich. Ocean salt water is full of minerals such as magnesium, zinc, iron, potassium, iodine, and sodium and has long been used to address a range of conditions. Immersion in or proximity to ocean waters can trigger any of these benefits to both body and mind:

- Improved and accelerated healing of wounds
- Relaxation
- The parasympathetic nervous system's rest-and-digest state
- Meditative state
- Reduced stress
- Quieting of the mind
- Blood oxygenation
- Relief of skin conditions like psoriasis or eczema
- Clarifying and cleansing

THE HEALING POWER OF THE PINEAL GLAND

OCEAN AIR-TO-SEA AWAKENING EXERCISE

Ready to dive in? Here's how to channel the ocean's calming energy to realign and recalibrate your third eye chakra.

- Head to the beach or any body of water, preferably before sunrise.

- Walk, run, bike, or simply sit in stillness while watching the sun rise over the sea and earth.

- Focus on the clarity of your breath. Feel each inhalation and exhalation. Observe the smells that fill your nostrils and the sounds that enter your ears.

- Enjoy the sensorial experience of the present moment, with daybreak bringing the promise of a new day, hope, and the feeling that anything is possible.

- If possible, return at sunset to the body of water or nature environment of your preference and repeat the exercise, watching the closing of the day.

- Breath in the gratitude of the moment, exhaling out anything you wish to release.

- Give yourself permission to be fully immersed in this moment to relax, release, and recalibrate your energy and aura. Acknowledge how your body feels, and observe your thoughts without judgment.

Summary

Whether you prefer the beach or the mountains, the land or sea, exploring and enjoying the natural wonders of the world improves our mood, shifts our perspective, and allows us to experience the energy of our natural surroundings. Even taking a different route on a daily walk or feeling anticipatory joy for an upcoming experience reenergizes the spirit and awakens positive energy.

CHAPTER 16

ENERGY-FLOW ACTIVATION EXERCISE

Blue Light Detox

> *"You leave old habits behind by starting out with the thought, 'I release the need for this in my life.'"*
>
> **—Wayne Dyer**

The majority of our exposure to blue light occurs during the day, from sunlight and artificial sources like television and computer screens. Blue light triggers the suppression of melatonin while stimulating the parts of our brain that create alertness. Blue light also elevates our heart rate and body temperature. These are helpful in improving attention and focus when properly timed during the daylight hours. Some studies even suggest that strategic exposure to blue light can help in the treatment of several sleep disorders.

This is helpful for cultivating attentiveness during the day, but blue light can have detrimental consequences in the evening, especially in the hours before bedtime. Evening exposure to blue light can mislead our brains into believing it's still daytime, making us feel alert, awake, and activated rather than relaxed and ready to move into rest.

Unlike much of humanity's history, when these rhythms were regulated by the natural progression of sunrise and sunset, we now live in a world often disrupted by artificial light. This disrupts our circadian rhythm and can cause an imbalance in the pineal gland and the third eye chakra.

Modern life is rife with advances in digital technology—and with these advances come distractions and other consequences. Between Zoom meetings, smartphones, and other computer uses, many of us spend significant time on our digital devices. Blue light emissions can interrupt our sleep and have negative effects on our eyesight. They can confuse the signals our brain and pineal gland receive about time of day, delaying production of the melatonin necessary for sleep.

Like all light, blue light is electromagnetic radiation, a usually invisible form of energy. The colors of light are interpreted by our eyes based on the amount of energy the light contains. A rainbow shows us the entire spectrum of visible light, while the light emitted by the sun is white light, a combination of all of the colors available in the visible light spectrum. Blue light, which is part of the invisible light spectrum, can negatively impair and affect several aspects of our well-being, such as alertness and hormone production, which includes that of the melatonin necessary to sleep both efficiently and productively.

While all types of visible light can affect circadian rhythms, the largest impacts are from blue light and sunlight. A 2011 Sleep in America poll by the National Sleep Foundation found that ninety percent of Americans report using an electronic device in the time before they go to sleep, often directly in their bed.[9] A decade later, it's quite possible these numbers have gone up.

These are some of the most common sources of artificial blue light:[10]

- Fluorescent lights
- LED lights
- Smartphones
- Televisions
- Computer screens
- Tablets
- E-readers
- Video game consoles

One of our goals in the evening hours should be to minimize the disruptive effects of blue light. The obvious solution? Turn off the sources of blue light! This is easier said than done for most of us, however, and may not be entirely possible. Below are some ideas to integrate into your daily and nightly routines to help reduce exposure to blue light that can be interrupting your sleep and interfering with your third eye chakra.

9. Rob Newsom, Sleep Foundation, "How Blue Light Affects Sleep," updated June 24, 2021, https://www.sleepfoundation.org/bedroom-environment/blue-light.

10. Michael Gradisar, Amy R. Wolfson, Allison G. Harvey, Lauren Hale, Russell Rosenberg, and Charles A. Czeisler, "The Sleep and Technology Use of Americans: Findings from the National Sleep Foundation's 2011 Sleep in America Poll," *Journal of Clinical Sleep Medicine* 9, no. 12: doi:10.5664/jcsm.3272.

BLUE LIGHT DETOX

- Wear glasses that block blue light.

- Dim, reduce, or eliminate LED and fluorescent lighting.

- Set a reminder or alarm to turn off unnecessary digital devices approximately two to three hours before bedtime.

- Choose a bedside lamp that uses light in the yellow or orange area of the spectrum.

- Adjust the settings on your smartphone, laptop, desktop computer, or tablet to "night mode" or "yellow light," which can reduce the amount of blue light emissions your eyes receive.

- Improve the environment you sleep in. If possible, banish digital devices from the bedroom completely. If that's not possible, or if there are light sources in your bedroom that don't turn off or dim, consider wearing a light-blocking eye mask while you snooze.

THE POWER DOWN HOUR

Another idea for a better night's sleep is this exercise from Dr. Michael Breus. Breus recommends the Power Down Hour, which allows you to finish your daily to-do's and get ready for sleep an hour before bedtime.

This exercise is carried out in three twenty-minute sessions.

- The first twenty minutes are reserved for taking care of simple, unfinished tasks such as light housework, pet care, tidying up, or taking out the trash.

- In the second block of twenty minutes, do something relaxing such as reading, playing music, doing a craft, journaling, meditating, or practicing an additional relaxation technique. Be careful not to turn to a screen during this time.

In the final twenty minutes, attend to your nighttime hygiene routine. Take a warm bath or shower, brush and floss your teeth, do any needed skincare, take out your contact lenses, and attend to any other bodily needs.

"Creating consistent and healthy rituals is key to getting a good night's sleep each night," says Dr. Breus. "And setting a specific time each evening to get things done is immensely helpful in making sure everything is taken care of at home and you get to bed on time."[11]

Summary

Maximize those precious moments before bed by eliminating—or minimizing—screen time and its corresponding, and potentially harmful, blue light emissions. By keeping digital devices out of the bedroom, you can protect your energy, and in turn, your peace, cultivating the calm, relaxed state of being needed to ease into an evening of fluid, healthy sleep.

---

11. Breus, Michael, PhD, American Board of Sleep Medicine Diplomate, American Academy of Sleep Medicine Fellow, Founder, www .thesleepdoctor.com. Phone interview and email correspondence, June and November 2021.

CONCLUSION

Thank you for joining me on this interactive journey to heal, detoxify, and unlock your pineal gland and third eye chakra. I hope these words, energy exercises, and holistic activities have brought newfound awareness, love, light, and activation into your life.

Our minds are magnetic forces of attraction, and our physical selves embody and emit energy that we share with the entire universe, including the one found within ourselves. As with anything we pursue, it takes continuously tapping into our minds and bodies to achieve the desired results.

As we moved through the activating activities in each chapter, we learned how to embody the energy within ourselves and emit it out into the world. By exploring the pineal gland and its intricacies, we learned how to work with it for optimum health. These mindful, meditative practices and energy-activating exercises allow us to treat, heal, and balance the elements of the mind, body, and spirit. Unlocking our own power allows us to create the shifts needed to expand into our fullest potential.

Continue to practice these energy-activating exercises with your whole heart, mind, and body. If you maintain your use of these exercises and activities, along with integrating other healthy habits into your daily life, you will recognize your own abilities to tap into your power. Use this book as a reference whenever you are feeling stuck—you'll be amazed at the creative spark of inspiration that will flow through your energetic field. Once you have awakened, elevated, and harnessed the energy and power of your pineal gland and third eye chakra, watch your newfound clarity and intuition elevate your life. Be aware and proud of your own power, and enjoy your newly empowered, activated, and fluidly energetic state of being!

APPENDIX

POSITIVE MORNING RITUAL

Try this ritual every morning. For an ongoing practice, make use of a separate notebook. Keep this book or the notebook on your nightstand so that you can easily access it without having to get up.

🖎 Write the phrase "I AM GRATEFUL" and list at least three things you feel gratitude for.

🖎 Next, write down the phrase "I AM MANIFESTING," "I AM INTENTIONAL," or "I AM DOING" and list the items you would like to integrate into your day.

🖎 Recite the lists aloud.

POSITIVE MORNING RITUAL

Try this ritual every morning. For an ongoing practice, make use of a separate notebook. Keep this book or the notebook on your nightstand so that you can easily access it without having to get up.

✎ Write the phrase "I AM GRATEFUL" and list at least three things you feel gratitude for.

✎ Next, write down the phrase "I AM MANIFESTING," "I AM INTENTIONAL," or "I AM DOING" and list the items you would like to integrate into your day.

✎ Recite the lists aloud.

POSITIVE MORNING RITUAL

Try this ritual every morning. For an ongoing practice, make use of a separate notebook. Keep this book or the notebook on your nightstand so that you can easily access it without having to get up.

≽ Write the phrase "I AM GRATEFUL" and list at least three things you feel gratitude for.

≽ Next, write down the phrase "I AM MANIFESTING," "I AM INTENTIONAL," or "I AM DOING" and list the items you would like to integrate into your day.

≽ Recite the lists aloud.

POSITIVE MORNING RITUAL

Try this ritual every morning. For an ongoing practice, make use of a separate notebook. Keep this book or the notebook on your nightstand so that you can easily access it without having to get up.

🖋 Write the phrase "I AM GRATEFUL" and list at least three things you feel gratitude for.

🖋 Next, write down the phrase "I AM MANIFESTING," "I AM INTENTIONAL," or "I AM DOING" and list the items you would like to integrate into your day.

🖋 Recite the lists aloud.

POSITIVE MORNING RITUAL

Try this ritual every morning. For an ongoing practice, make use of a separate notebook. Keep this book or the notebook on your nightstand so that you can easily access it without having to get up.

✎ Write the phrase "I AM GRATEFUL" and list at least three things you feel gratitude for.

✎ Next, write down the phrase "I AM MANIFESTING," "I AM INTENTIONAL," or "I AM DOING" and list the items you would like to integrate into your day.

✎ Recite the lists aloud.

EVENING AFFIRMATIONS

Perform these affirmations prior to bedtime in order to allow them to be fully absorbed into your subconscious as you sleep.

- Write the phrase "Amazing Things That Happened Today" and list three (or more) of the day's activities or happenings that made you feel grateful. It just might make you smile to relive these events and their joyful emotions!

- Write the phrase "I AM MANIFESTING" or "I AM INTENT ON" and beneath it list items you'd like to put into action.

- Place this book on your nightstand or next to your pillow to harness the power of subconscious thought manifesting into action.

EVENING AFFIRMATIONS

Perform these affirmations prior to bedtime in order to allow them to be fully absorbed into your subconscious as you sleep.

- Write the phrase "Amazing Things That Happened Today" and list three (or more) of the day's activities or happenings that made you feel grateful. It just might make you smile to relive these events and their joyful emotions!

- Write the phrase "I AM MANIFESTING" or "I AM INTENT ON" and beneath it list items you'd like to put into action.

- Place this book on your nightstand or next to your pillow to harness the power of subconscious thought manifesting into action.

EVENING AFFIRMATIONS

Perform these affirmations prior to bedtime in order to allow them to be fully absorbed into your subconscious as you sleep.

🖎 Write the phrase "Amazing Things That Happened Today" and list three (or more) of the day's activities or happenings that made you feel grateful. It just might make you smile to relive these events and their joyful emotions!

🖎 Write the phrase "I AM MANIFESTING" or "I AM INTENT ON" and beneath it list items you'd like to put into action.

🖎 Place this book on your nightstand or next to your pillow to harness the power of subconscious thought manifesting into action.

EVENING AFFIRMATIONS

Perform these affirmations prior to bedtime in order to allow them to be fully absorbed into your subconscious as you sleep.

- ✎ Write the phrase "Amazing Things That Happened Today" and list three (or more) of the day's activities or happenings that made you feel grateful. It just might make you smile to relive these events and their joyful emotions!

- ✎ Write the phrase "I AM MANIFESTING" or "I AM INTENT ON" and beneath it list items you'd like to put into action.

- ✎ Place this book on your nightstand or next to your pillow to harness the power of subconscious thought manifesting into action.

EVENING AFFIRMATIONS

Perform these affirmations prior to bedtime in order to allow them to be fully absorbed into your subconscious as you sleep.

- ✍ Write the phrase "Amazing Things That Happened Today" and list three (or more) of the day's activities or happenings that made you feel grateful. It just might make you smile to relive these events and their joyful emotions!

- ✍ Write the phrase "I AM MANIFESTING" or "I AM INTENT ON" and beneath it list items you'd like to put into action.

- ✍ Place this book on your nightstand or next to your pillow to harness the power of subconscious thought manifesting into action.

WORKS CITED

Breus, Michael. Phone interview and email correspondence. June and November 2021.

Easwaran, Eknath. *The Upanishads*. 2nd Edition. Tomales, CA: Nilgiri Press, 2007.

Easwaran, Eknath. *The Bhagavad Gita*. 2nd Edition. Tomales, CA: Nilgiri Press, 2007.

Emmons, Robert A., and Michael E. McCullough. "Counting Blessing Versus Burdens: An Experimental Investigation of Gratitude and Subjective Well-Being in Daily Life." *Journal of Personality and Social Psychology* 84, no. 2 (February 2003): 377–89. Doi.org/10.1037/0022-3514.84.2.377.

Gradisar, Michael, Amy R. Wolfson, Allison G. Harvey, Lauren Hale, Russell Rosenberg, and Charles A. Czeisler. "The Sleep and Technology Use of Americans: Findings from the National Sleep Foundation's 2011 Sleep in America Poll." *Journal of Clinical Sleep Medicine* 9, no. 12 (December 2015): 1291–9. Doi.org/10.5664/jcsm.3272.

Hall, Judy. *The Crystal Seer: Power Crystals for Magic, Meditation, & Ritual*. Beverly, MA: Fair Winds Press Inc., 2018.

Hartranft, Chip. *The Yoga-Sutra of Patanjali: Shambhala*. Boulder, CO: Shambala Publications, 2003.

Iyengar, B.K.S. *Core of the Yoga Sutras: The Definitive Guide to the Philosophy of Yoga*. New York: Harper Thorsons, 2013.

Iyengar, B. K. S. *Light on Yoga: The Bible of Modern Yoga*. Crows Nest, Australia: Allen & Unwin, 1965.

Iyengar, B.K.S. *Light on Yoga: The Bible of Modern Yoga*. New York: Schocken Books, 2006.

Meng, Xiao, Ya Li, Sha Li, Yue Zhou, Ren-You Gan, Dong-Ping Xu, and Hua-Bin Li. "Dietary Sources and Bioactivities of Melatonin." *Nutrients* 9, no. 4 (2017): 367. Doi.org/10.339/nu9040367.

Newsom, Rob. "How Blue Light Affects Sleep." Sleep Foundation. Last updated June 24, 2021. https://www.sleepfoundation.org/bedroom-environment/blue-light.

Patañjali, and Alistair Shearer. *The Yoga Sutras of Patanjali*. New York: Harmony Books, 2002.

Perrakis, PhD., Athena. *Crystal Lore, Legends & Myths*. Beverly, MA: Quarto Publishing Group USA Inc., 2019.

Satchidananda, Sri Swami. *The Yoga Sutras of Patanjali*. Buckingham, VA: Integral Yoga Publications, 2012.

WebMD. "What to Know About Calcification of the Pineal Gland." Last updated June 23, 2021. https://www.webmd.com/sleep-disorders/what-to-know-about-calcification-of-the-pineal-gland.

Yoga for the Conception Journey. "Many Believe Meditation is Practiced Simply to Clear the Mind." Facebook, August 4, 2021. https://www.facebook.com/hashtag/yogaforttc?source=feed_text&epa=HASHTAG.

Mead, Olivia. Email message and interview with author. May 2021.

Oschman, James L., Gaetan Chevalier, and Richard Brown. "The Effects of Grounding (Earthing) on Inflammation, the Immune Response, Wound Healing, and Prevention and Treatment of Chronic Inflammatory and Autoimmune Diseases." *Journal of Inflammation Research* 8, (March 2015): 83–96. Doi.org/10.2147/JIR.S69656.

Upanishads. Translated by F. Max-Muller. Hertfordshire, UK: Wordsworth Editions Limited, 2001.

Zaraska, Marta. "The Sense of Smell in Humans Is More Powerful Than We Think." *Discover Magazine*. October 10, 2017. https://www.discovermagazine.com/mind/the-sense-of-smell-in-humans-is-more -powerful-than-we-think.

ACKNOWLEDGMENTS

I have long been a believer in divine timing and the law of attraction—so much so that when the opportunity to write this book presented itself, I felt it was truly a gift. It was the sign I needed from the universe that things were unfolding as they were meant to, and that I was exactly where I needed to be.

With that being said, I am also grateful to share these mindful practices. I hope that they have brought—and will continue to bring—light, love, and consciousness to you in a similar manner in which they have provided solace for me.

I would also like to thank my loved ones, especially my parents, for their support and encouragement, not only during the writing process, but throughout all the years leading up to this work. I am grateful for all those who have supported, encouraged, and read the words I have written over the years. To my yoga students, thank you for showing up with energy, devotion, and, most of all, giving me the opportunity to continue the process of evolution. In yoga and in life, we are always students, learning, adapting, flowing, and seeking to bring our minds and bodies into balance, seamlessly moving into a place of ease, expansion, openness, lightness, and peace.

Finally, thank you readers for coming on this journey with me. I am so grateful to share positive energy and these mindful practices, and I'm excited for your path to unfold, evolve, and expand. Namaste!

ABOUT THE AUTHOR

Crystal Fenton is a freelance writer and E-RYT®200 YACEP® certified Yoga Instructor. As a multimedia journalist, her editorial work has appeared in numerous print and digital magazines and television outlets, covering yoga, wellness, health, meditation, science, lifestyle, beauty, travel, and more.

As a yoga and meditation instructor, her work includes private and semiprivate teaching at workshops, events, and group sessions. She has been a panel speaker and provided expertise on working with active and retired first responders, including firefighters, military and law enforcement personnel, professional athletes, cancer patients and patients with other serious illness, and other trauma-informed populations.

The Healing Power of the Pineal Gland: Exercises and Meditations to Detoxify, Decalcify, and Activate Your Third Eye is her first book.